WORKOUT

and

EXERCISE PLAN

for beginners

A Beginner's Roadmap to Strength,
Resilience, and Radiant Health

RICHARD L. LYONS

TABLE OF CONTENT

INTRODUCTION

Welcome, and congratulations on taking the first step towards a healthier, more vibrant lifestyle! The decision to embark on a fitness journey is a powerful one, and it's a testament to your commitment to prioritizing your overall well-being. Whether you're seeking to improve your physical health, boost your energy levels, or simply feel better about yourself, you've made a wise choice in exploring the world of exercise and physical activity.

In today's fast-paced and sedentary world, it's all too easy to neglect the importance of movement and exercise. We spend countless hours glued to our screens, hunched over desks, and confined within the four walls of our homes or offices. However, this inactive lifestyle comes at a significant cost to our health, both physically and mentally. Regular exercise is not only crucial for maintaining a healthy weight and reducing the risk of chronic diseases but also plays a vital role in enhancing our mood, reducing stress and anxiety, and improving sleep quality.

The benefits of exercise and physical activity are far-reaching and profound. From a physical standpoint, regular exercise can help to strengthen our muscles, improve cardiovascular health, increase flexibility and range of motion, and boost our metabolism. It can also play a crucial role in managing and preventing a wide range of health conditions, including obesity, type 2 diabetes, high blood pressure, and certain types of cancer.

But the advantages of exercise extend far beyond the physical realm. Regular physical activity has been shown to have a positive impact on mental health and overall well-being. Exercise releases endorphins, which are natural mood-boosters, and can help alleviate symptoms of depression and anxiety. It can also improve cognitive function, enhance focus and concentration, and boost self-esteem and body image.

Perhaps most importantly, exercise has the power to improve our overall quality of life. By prioritizing physical activity, we can experience increased energy levels, better sleep, improved stamina, and a greater sense of accomplishment and self-confidence. Exercise can also serve as a powerful tool for stress management, providing a healthy outlet for releasing tension and clearing our minds.

With this book, "Workout and Exercise Plan for Beginners," we aim to guide you through the exciting and transformative world of exercise, empowering you to take control of your health and well-being. Within these pages, you'll find a wealth of information, practical tips, and detailed workout routines designed specifically for those new to the fitness journey.

We'll start by exploring the importance of setting realistic and achievable goals, as well as creating a balanced workout plan that incorporates various types of exercise, including cardiovascular activities, strength training, flexibility work, and more. We'll delve into the art of warm-up and stretching exercises, ensuring that you're properly prepared for your workouts and minimizing the risk of injury.

From there, we'll dive into the world of cardiovascular exercise, exploring a variety of activities that can help improve your heart health, boost your endurance, and aid in weight management. We'll also provide you with a comprehensive guide to upper and lower body strength training, equipping you with the knowledge and techniques to build lean muscle mass, increase bone density, and enhance overall strength and power.

But exercise is about more than just cardio and strength training. We'll explore the importance of core strengthening exercises, which can help improve your posture, balance, and overall stability, as well as flexibility and mobility exercises that can enhance your range of motion and reduce the risk of injury.

For those seeking a more intense and efficient workout, we'll introduce you to the world of High-Intensity Interval Training (HIIT), a powerful technique that combines bursts of intense exercise with periods of rest, allowing you to maximize your calorie burn and cardiovascular benefits in a shorter amount of time.

As you progress on your fitness journey, we'll guide you through the principles of progressive overload and progressive resistance, ensuring that you continue to challenge yourself and achieve consistent progress towards your goals. We'll also provide you with a range of workout routines tailored to specific goals, whether you're aiming for weight loss, muscle gain, improved endurance, or overall fitness.

But physical exercise is only one piece of the puzzle. We understand the importance of a well-rounded approach to health and well-being, which is why we've dedicated an entire chapter to nutrition and supplementation. We'll provide you with practical tips and strategies for fueling your body with the nutrients it needs to support your workout routine, recover properly, and achieve optimal performance.

Rest and recovery are equally important components of a successful fitness program, and we'll explore various techniques and strategies to help you maximize your recovery and avoid overtraining or injury. We'll also address common mistakes and injuries that often plague beginners, equipping you with the knowledge and tools to exercise safely and effectively.

Throughout this book, we'll emphasize the importance of staying motivated and consistent, offering practical tips and strategies for overcoming obstacles, celebrating milestones, and maintaining a positive and dedicated mindset throughout your fitness journey. We understand that consistency is key to achieving long-term success, and we'll provide you with the tools and resources you need to stay on track and continue making progress.

By the end of this book, you'll not only have a comprehensive understanding of the various components of a well-rounded fitness program but also the knowledge and confidence to create and implement a personalized workout and exercise plan that aligns with your unique goals, preferences, and lifestyle.

Remember, the journey towards a healthier, more active lifestyle is a marathon, not a sprint. It's a lifelong commitment to prioritizing your well-being and embracing the transformative power of movement and exercise. With dedication, patience, and a willingness to learn and grow, you'll be well on your way to unlocking a whole new world of physical and mental vitality.

So, let's embark on this exciting adventure together. Turn the page, and let's begin your journey towards a stronger, healthier, and more vibrant you!

CHAPTER 1

SETTING GOALS AND CREATING A WORKOUT PLAN

As you embark on your fitness journey, one of the most critical steps is setting clear, achievable goals and creating a well-structured workout plan. Without a roadmap and a destination in mind, it's all too easy to lose motivation and veer off course. In this chapter, we'll explore the importance of goal-setting, discuss how to craft realistic and attainable fitness objectives, and provide you with the tools and strategies to develop a comprehensive workout plan tailored to your unique needs and preferences.

The Power Of Goal-setting

Goals are powerful motivators that can help us stay focused, accountable, and driven towards our desired outcomes. When it comes to fitness, setting goals can serve as a compass, guiding us through the often-challenging journey of lifestyle changes and physical transformation.

Well-defined goals not only provide us with a clear target to work towards but also offer a sense of purpose and direction. They enable us to measure our progress, celebrate milestones, and make adjustments along the way. Without goals, it's easy to feel aimless and discouraged, which can quickly derail even the most well-intentioned fitness efforts.

Crafting Realistic and Achievable Fitness Goals

While the importance of goal-setting is undeniable, it's equally crucial to ensure that your goals are realistic and achievable. Setting overly ambitious or unrealistic targets can lead to frustration, disappointment, and ultimately, a loss of motivation.

When defining your fitness goals, it's essential to consider your current fitness level, lifestyle constraints, and personal preferences. For example, if you're new to exercise, setting a goal of running a marathon within the next three months may be unrealistic and could set you up for failure. Instead, focus on smaller, more achievable milestones, such as gradually increasing your weekly exercise frequency or completing a 5K race within a reasonable timeframe.

One effective approach to goal-setting is the SMART method, which stands for Specific, Measurable, Achievable, Relevant, and Time-bound. Let's break down each component:

- **Specific**: Your goals should be clear and well-defined, leaving no room for ambiguity. Instead of setting a vague goal like "getting in shape," aim for something more precise, such as "losing

10 pounds" or "increasing my bench press by 20 pounds."

- **Measurable**: Quantifiable goals allow you to track your progress and celebrate milestones along the way. For example, "exercise for 30 minutes, five days a week" or "run a mile without stopping" are measurable goals that provide a clear benchmark for success.

- **Achievable**: While it's important to challenge yourself, your goals should also be realistic and attainable given your current circumstances and limitations. Setting overly ambitious goals can quickly lead to discouragement and a loss of motivation.

- **Relevant**: Your fitness goals should align with your broader life goals and personal values. If your objective is to improve your overall health and well-being, a goal of completing an ultramarathon may not be the most relevant or practical choice.

- **Time-bound**: Attaching a specific timeframe to your goals can help create a sense of urgency and accountability. For example, "lose 10 pounds in three months" or "complete a 5K race by the end of the summer."

By following the SMART framework, you can ensure that your fitness goals are well-defined, measurable, achievable, relevant, and time-bound, increasing your chances of success and long-term commitment.

Understanding Different Types Of Workouts

Once you've established your fitness goals, the next step is to understand the various types of workouts and how they can contribute to your overall fitness and well-being. A balanced and well-rounded workout routine should incorporate a combination of cardiovascular exercise, strength training, and flexibility work.

Cardiovascular Exercise:

Cardiovascular exercise, also known as aerobic exercise, is any activity that increases your heart rate and breathing rate for an extended period. This type of exercise is crucial for improving cardiovascular health, boosting endurance, and aiding in weight management. Examples of cardiovascular exercises include:

- Running or jogging
- Cycling
- Swimming
- Rowing
- Jumping rope
- High-intensity interval training (HIIT)

Strength Training:

Strength training, or resistance training, involves the use of weights, resistance bands, or your own body weight to build muscle strength and endurance. This type of exercise is essential for increasing lean muscle mass, improving bone density, and boosting metabolism. Strength training can be further divided into upper body and lower body exercises:

Upper Body Exercises:

- Push-ups
- Pull-ups
- Bicep curls
- Tricep dips
- Shoulder presses

Lower Body Exercises:

- Squats
- Lunges
- Deadlifts
- Calf raises
- Step-ups

Flexibility and Mobility:

Flexibility and mobility exercises are often overlooked but are crucial components of a well-rounded fitness routine. These exercises help improve your range of motion, reduce the risk of injury, and promote overall physical functionality. Examples of flexibility and mobility exercises include:

- Static stretching
- Dynamic stretching
- Foam rolling
- Yoga
- Pilates

Creating a Balanced Routine

To maximize the benefits of your workout routine and achieve your fitness goals, it's essential to incorporate a combination of cardiovascular exercise, strength training, and flexibility work. A balanced routine not only ensures that you're targeting all aspects of physical fitness but also helps prevent overuse injuries and promotes overall body balance.

Here's an example of a well-rounded weekly workout routine:

Monday: Full-body strength training

Tuesday: Cardiovascular exercise (e.g., running or cycling)

Wednesday: Rest or active recovery (e.g., yoga or light stretching)

Thursday: Lower body strength training and core work

Friday: Cardiovascular exercise (e.g., HIIT or swimming)

Saturday: Upper body strength training

Sunday: Rest or active recovery (e.g., hiking or walking)

Remember, this is just an example, and your specific routine should be tailored to your individual goals, preferences, and schedule. The key is to find a balance that works for you and to consistently challenge yourself while allowing for adequate rest and recovery.

Tips for Scheduling Workouts and Staying Motivated

While setting goals and creating a workout plan are essential first steps, the real challenge often lies in consistently adhering to your routine and maintaining your motivation over time. Here are some tips to help you stay on track:

1. **Schedule your workouts**: Treat your workout sessions like important appointments and schedule them in advance. Blocking off dedicated time in your calendar can help ensure that exercise remains a priority amidst the demands of daily life.

2. **Find a workout buddy**: Having an exercise partner can make your workouts more enjoyable and provide an added layer of accountability. Workout buddies can offer encouragement, friendly competition, and a shared commitment to your fitness goals.

3. **Mix it up**: Variety is the spice of life, and the same principle applies to your workout routine. Mixing up your exercises, trying new activities, or varying the intensity can help prevent boredom and keep you engaged and motivated.

4. **Set reminders**: Utilize technology to your advantage by setting reminders or alarms on your smartphone, smartwatch, or calendar to prompt you to exercise at your scheduled times.

5. **Track your progress**: Keeping a workout log or using a fitness tracking app can help you monitor your progress, celebrate milestones, and stay motivated by visualizing your achievements over time.

6. **Reward yourself**: Set small, achievable milestones and reward yourself when you reach them. These rewards can be non-food-related

treats, such as a new workout outfit, a massage, or a night out with friends.

7. **Find your "why"**: Reconnect with your deeper motivations for pursuing a healthier lifestyle. Whether it's to have more energy for your family, reduce the risk of chronic diseases, or improve your self-confidence, reminding yourself of your "why" can provide the necessary fuel to power through challenging moments.

8. **Be patient and persistent**: Remember that true, lasting change takes time and consistency. There will be setbacks and plateaus along the way, but staying patient and persistent will ultimately yield the desired results.

By incorporating these strategies into your fitness routine, you'll be better equipped to overcome obstacles, maintain your motivation, and stay committed to your workout plan, bringing you one step closer to achieving your fitness goals.

Remember, setting goals and creating a workout plan is just the beginning of your fitness journey. The real challenge lies in consistently showing up, pushing yourself, and embracing the transformative power of exercise. With dedication, patience, and a well-rounded approach, you'll be on your way to unlocking a healthier, more vibrant version of yourself.

CHAPTER 2

WARM-UP AND STRETCHING EXERCISES

As you embark on your fitness journey, it's essential to understand the importance of properly preparing your body for physical activity. Warm-up and stretching exercises are often overlooked, but they play a crucial role in injury prevention, improving flexibility, and optimizing performance. In this chapter, we'll delve into the science behind warm-ups and stretching, explore the benefits of incorporating these practices into your routine, and provide you with a comprehensive guide to dynamic warm-up exercises and static stretches for major muscle groups.

The Importance Of Warm-ups and Stretching

Warm-ups and stretching are not merely optional extras but rather vital components of a well-rounded fitness routine. These preparatory exercises serve several important functions:

1. **Injury Prevention**:

One of the primary benefits of warm-ups and stretching is their ability to reduce the risk of injury. When you engage in physical activity without properly preparing your muscles, tendons, and joints, you increase the likelihood of strains, sprains, and other injuries. Warm-ups gradually raise your body temperature, increase blood flow, and lubricate your joints, making your muscles more pliable and less susceptible to injury.

2. **Increased Flexibility**:

Stretching exercises are designed to improve your range of motion and flexibility. As we age, our muscles and connective tissues naturally become tighter and less elastic, which can limit our mobility and increase the risk of injury. Regular stretching can help counteract this process, allowing you to maintain and even enhance your flexibility, which is essential for performing various exercises and everyday activities with ease.

3. **Enhanced Performance**:

By properly warming up and preparing your muscles for the demands of your workout, you can optimize your performance and potentially achieve better results. Warm muscles are more responsive, allowing for greater power generation, improved coordination, and increased endurance during your exercise sessions.

4. **Mental Preparation**:

In addition to the physical benefits, warm-ups and stretching can also help mentally prepare you for your workout. These preparatory exercises can serve as a transition period, allowing you to shift your focus from the stresses of daily life to the task at hand, promoting a more mindful and present approach to your training.

Dynamic warm-up exercises are designed to gradually increase your heart rate, body temperature, and range of motion. These active movements mimic the specific motions you'll perform during your workout, preparing your muscles and joints for the upcoming physical demands. Here are some examples of effective dynamic warm-up exercises:

1. **Jogging or Marching in Place**:

This simple exercise helps raise your heart rate and increase blood flow throughout your body.

2. **High Knees**:

Bring your knees up toward your chest, one at a time, while pumping your arms. This exercise warms up your hip flexors and gets your heart rate elevated.

3. **Butt Kicks**:

Similar to high knees, but instead of bringing your knees up, you'll kick your heels toward your glutes, alternating legs. This exercise targets your hamstrings and glutes.

4. Arm Circles:

Rotate your arms in a circular motion, both forwards and backwards, to warm up your shoulder joints and surrounding muscles.

5. Leg Swings:

Stand with one hand on a wall for support, and gently swing your leg forward and backward, and then side to side. This exercise helps increase mobility in your hip joints and prepare your legs for more dynamic movements.

6. Jumping Jacks:

This classic exercise gets your heart rate up while also warming up your entire body and improving coordination.

7. **Lunges**:

Step forward with one leg, lowering your hips toward the ground, and then repeat on the other side. Lunges are a great way to warm up your lower body, particularly your quadriceps, hamstrings, and glutes.

Remember, the key to an effective dynamic warm-up is to start slowly and gradually increase the intensity and range of motion. These exercises should be performed in a controlled manner, without bouncing or jerking movements, to avoid injury.

Static Stretches for Major Muscle Groups

After completing your dynamic warm-up, it's time to move on to static stretching. Static stretches are designed to lengthen and elongate specific muscle groups, improving flexibility and range of motion. Here are examples of effective static stretches targeting major muscle groups:

1. **Hamstring Stretches:**

- Seated Forward Fold: Sit on the floor with your legs extended in front of you. Reach forward, keeping your back straight, and gently fold over your legs, reaching toward your toes.

- Standing Hamstring Stretch: Stand with one leg elevated on a bench or chair. Keeping your back straight, hinge forward at the hips, reaching your hands toward your elevated foot.

2. **Quadriceps Stretches:**

- Standing Quad Stretch: Stand with one hand on a wall for balance. Bend one knee and grab your ankle or foot, gently pulling your heel toward your glutes.

- Kneeling Quad Stretch: Kneel on one knee, with your other leg extended in front of you. Keeping your upper body upright, lean back, feeling the stretch in the front of your thigh.

3. **Calf Stretches**:

- Wall Calf Stretch: Stand facing a wall, with your hands against the wall at shoulder height. Step back with one leg, keeping your heel on the ground, and lean forward to feel the stretch in your calf.

- Runner's Calf Stretch: In a split stance, with one leg forward and one leg back, bend your front knee and lean forward, keeping your back heel on the ground.

4. **Hip Flexor Stretches**:

- Kneeling Hip Flexor Stretch: Kneel on one knee, with your other leg extended in front of you, foot flat on the floor. Gently lean your hips forward, keeping your upper body upright, to feel the stretch in the front of your hip.

- Butterfly Stretch: Sit on the floor with the soles of your feet together, knees bent outward.

Gently press down on your knees with your elbows to deepen the stretch in your inner thighs and groin area.

5. **Upper Body Stretches**:

- Overhead Triceps Stretch: Raise one arm overhead and bend your elbow, reaching your hand down between your shoulder blades. Use your other hand to gently pull the stretching arm closer to your head.

- Chest Stretch: Stand in a doorway or corner, with your arms extended and hands at shoulder height on the walls or doorframe. Step forward with one leg, feeling the stretch across your chest and shoulders.

Remember, when performing static stretches, it's important to hold each stretch for at least 15-30 seconds, breathing deeply and avoiding bouncing or jerking movements. If you feel any sharp pain or discomfort, ease off the stretch or stop altogether.

Incorporating Warm-Ups and Stretching into Your Routine

Now that you understand the importance of warm-ups and stretching, as well as the specific exercises to include, it's time to incorporate these practices into your overall fitness routine. Here are some tips to help you get started:

1. **Allocate Time:**

Set aside 10-15 minutes before your workout to complete a dynamic warm-up and static stretching routine. This dedicated time will ensure that you properly prepare your body for the upcoming physical demands.

2. **Tailor Your Routine:**

While the exercises provided in this chapter are excellent starting points, feel free to customize your warm-up and stretching routine to suit your specific needs and preferences. If you have areas of tightness or limited mobility, focus on stretches that target those muscle groups.

3. **Listen to Your Body**:

Pay attention to how your body feels during and after your warm-up and stretching routine. If you experience any pain or discomfort, adjust or stop the exercise immediately. Remember, the goal is to prepare your body, not cause injury.

4. **Consistency is Key**:

Make warm-ups and stretching a non-negotiable part of your fitness routine. Consistency is crucial for reaping the full benefits of these preparatory exercises and developing a habit that will serve you well in the long run.

5. **Incorporate Active Recovery**:

On your rest or active recovery days, consider incorporating additional stretching and mobility exercises to promote muscle recovery and maintain flexibility. Techniques like foam rolling, yoga, or Pilates can be excellent options.

By prioritizing warm-ups and stretching, you'll not only reduce your risk of injury but also optimize your performance and overall exercise experience. Remember, taking the time to properly prepare your body is an investment in your long-term health and fitness journey.

CHAPTER 3

CARDIOVASCULAR EXERCISES

At the heart of any well-rounded fitness program lies cardiovascular exercise, a powerful tool that can profoundly impact your overall health and well-being. Often referred to as "cardio," these activities engage your heart, lungs, and circulatory system, providing a wealth of benefits that extend far beyond physical appearance. In this chapter, we'll delve into the science behind cardiovascular exercise, explore its numerous advantages, and provide you with a comprehensive guide to various cardio modalities, ensuring you have the knowledge and resources to incorporate this crucial component into your workout routine effectively.

Understanding Cardiovascular Exercise

Cardiovascular exercise, or aerobic exercise, refers to any physical activity that elevates your heart rate and breathing rate for an extended period. During these activities, your body relies primarily on aerobic metabolism, which utilizes oxygen to produce energy. This process not only challenges your cardiovascular system but also engages multiple muscle groups, leading to a host of physiological benefits.

The Benefits of Cardiovascular Exercise

Incorporating regular cardiovascular exercise into your lifestyle can yield numerous advantages, positively impacting various aspects of your health and well-being:

1. **Improved Cardiovascular Health:**

Regular cardio workouts strengthen your heart muscle, improving its ability to pump blood more efficiently throughout your body. This, in turn, can lower your resting heart rate, reduce blood pressure levels, and decrease your risk of developing heart disease, stroke, and other cardiovascular conditions.

2. **Enhanced Respiratory Function:**

Cardiovascular exercise improves the efficiency of your lungs, increasing their capacity to take in oxygen and expel carbon dioxide. This enhanced respiratory function can lead to improved endurance and overall breathing capacity, benefiting individuals with respiratory conditions like asthma or COPD.

3. **Weight Management:**

Cardio exercises are excellent for burning calories and aiding in weight loss or maintenance. By engaging large muscle groups and elevating your heart rate, you can significantly increase your caloric expenditure during and after your workout, helping to create the calorie deficit necessary for weight loss.

4. **Increased Endurance and Stamina:**

Regular cardiovascular training helps improve your body's ability to deliver oxygen to working muscles, enabling you to perform physical activities for more extended periods without fatigue. This increased endurance and stamina can benefit you in various aspects of your life, from participating in recreational activities to tackling daily tasks with greater ease.

5. **Improved Mood and Mental Health**:

Cardiovascular exercise has been shown to stimulate the release of endorphins, the body's natural mood-boosting chemicals. Regular cardio workouts can help alleviate symptoms of depression, anxiety, and stress, while also improving self-esteem and overall mental well-being.

6. **Reduced Risk of Chronic Diseases**:

By maintaining a healthy weight, lowering blood pressure, and improving insulin sensitivity, regular cardiovascular exercise can significantly reduce your risk of developing chronic conditions such as type 2 diabetes, certain types of cancer, and metabolic disorders.

With a broad understanding of the benefits of cardiovascular exercise, it's time to explore the various modalities available to you. The beauty of cardio lies in the vast array of options, ensuring there's something to suit every preference, fitness level, and lifestyle:

1. **Running/Jogging**:

One of the most popular and accessible forms of cardio, running or jogging can be done virtually anywhere, requiring minimal equipment. Whether you prefer hitting the pavement, treadmill, or trail, this high-impact activity provides an excellent cardiovascular challenge while also strengthening your bones and muscles.

2. **Cycling**:

Cycling is a low-impact cardio option that's gentle on your joints while still providing an effective workout for your cardiovascular system. You can cycle outdoors, exploring scenic routes or indoor on a stationary bike, making it a versatile choice for all seasons and weather conditions.

3. **Swimming**:

For those seeking a full-body, low-impact workout, swimming is an excellent choice. This aquatic activity engages multiple muscle groups while providing resistance, making it an effective cardiovascular exercise that's also gentle on your joints.

4. **Rowing**:

Rowing combines the benefits of cardiovascular exercise with strength training, targeting your legs, core, and upper body. You can row on the water or use an indoor rowing machine, providing a challenging, full-body workout that can be tailored to your fitness level.

5. **Jumping Rope**:

Don't underestimate the power of this simple childhood activity. Jumping rope is an incredibly effective cardio exercise that can be performed virtually anywhere, making it a convenient and inexpensive option for those short on time or space.

6. **High-Intensity Interval Training (HIIT)**:

HIIT involves short bursts of intense exercise followed by periods of rest or lower-intensity recovery. This time-efficient approach can provide significant cardiovascular benefits while also boosting your metabolism and promoting fat loss.

7. **Dancing**:

Whether you prefer structured dance classes or simply moving to your favorite tunes at home, dancing is an enjoyable and creative way to get your heart rate up. From salsa and Zumba to hip-hop and ballet, there's a dance style to suit every taste and preference.

8. **Sports and Recreational Activities:**

Engaging in sports or recreational activities like basketball, tennis, soccer, or even hiking can provide an excellent cardiovascular workout while adding an element of fun and social interaction to your fitness routine.

Tips for Incorporating Cardio into Your Workout Routine

Now that you have a comprehensive understanding of cardiovascular exercise and its various modalities, it's time to integrate it into your workout routine effectively. Here are some tips to help you get started:

1. **Set Realistic Goals:**

Start by setting achievable goals for your cardio workouts, considering your current fitness level, schedule, and preferences. For beginners, aim for at least 150 minutes of moderate-intensity cardio or 75 minutes of vigorous-intensity cardio per week, gradually increasing as you build endurance.

2. **Mix It Up:**

To prevent boredom and challenge your body in different ways, try incorporating a variety of cardio exercises into your routine. This can help prevent plateaus and keep you motivated while targeting different muscle groups and energy systems.

3. **Incorporate Intervals**:

Adding intervals, or periods of higher intensity followed by recovery periods, can help you maximize the benefits of your cardio workouts. HIIT sessions can be an effective way to boost your metabolism, improve endurance, and promote fat loss in a shorter amount of time.

4. **Listen to Your Body:**

While pushing yourself is important for progress, it's equally crucial to listen to your body's signals. If you feel excessively fatigued, experience pain, or struggle to catch your breath, it's okay to scale back or take a rest day.

5. **Stay Hydrated**:

Cardiovascular exercise can lead to significant fluid loss through sweating, so it's essential to stay hydrated before, during, and after your workouts. Carry a water bottle with you and sip regularly to replenish lost fluids.

6. **Cross-Train**:

Incorporate other forms of exercise, such as strength training and flexibility work, into your routine to create a well-rounded fitness program. Cross-training can help prevent overuse injuries, improve overall fitness, and keep your workouts interesting and engaging.

7. **Find Activities You Enjoy:**

While all cardio exercises offer benefits, it's essential to find activities you genuinely enjoy. When you look forward to your workouts, you're more likely to stick with them consistently, increasing the chances of achieving your fitness goals.

8.   **Track Your Progress**:

Regularly track your cardio workouts, noting the duration, intensity, and any improvements or milestones achieved. This can help you stay motivated, identify areas for improvement, and adjust your routine as needed.

Remember, consistency is key when it comes to reaping the full benefits of cardiovascular exercise. By incorporating cardio into your routine and gradually increasing the duration and intensity, you'll be well on your way to improving your overall health, fitness, and quality of life.

CHAPTER 4

UPPER BODY STRENGTH TRAINING

In the pursuit of a well-rounded and effective fitness routine, strength training is an essential component that can no longer be overlooked. While cardiovascular exercise is crucial for heart health and endurance, strength training plays a vital role in building lean muscle mass, increasing bone density, and boosting overall strength and functional ability. In this chapter, we'll delve into the importance of strength training, explore its numerous benefits, and provide you with a comprehensive guide to upper body exercises and proper form, equipping you with the knowledge and tools to incorporate this powerful aspect of fitness into your routine.

Strength training, also known as resistance training, involves the use of external resistance to challenge your muscles and stimulate growth. This resistance can come in the form of weights, resistance bands, or even your own body weight. By consistently exposing your muscles to this stress, they are forced to adapt and become stronger, leading to a host of physical and mental benefits:

1. **Increased Muscle Mass:**

One of the most evident benefits of strength training is the development of lean muscle mass. As you challenge your muscles with resistance, they are stimulated to grow and become stronger, leading to improved definition and overall body composition.

2. **Enhanced Bone Density:**

The stress placed on your bones during strength training exercises helps to stimulate the formation of new bone tissue, increasing bone density and reducing the risk of osteoporosis and age-related fractures.

3. **Boosted Metabolism:**

Muscle tissue is metabolically active, meaning it requires more energy (calories) to maintain itself compared to fat tissue. By increasing your muscle mass through strength training, you can effectively boost your resting metabolic rate, making it easier to manage your weight and body composition.

4. **Improved Functional Strength:**

Strength training can enhance your ability to perform daily tasks with greater ease, from carrying groceries and lifting heavy objects to climbing stairs and participating in recreational activities. This improved functional strength can contribute to a higher quality of life and increased independence as you age.

5. **Better Posture and Balance:**

By targeting and strengthening the muscles responsible for maintaining proper posture and balance, strength training can help improve your overall stability and coordination, reducing the risk of falls and injuries.

6.   **Increased Confidence and Self-Esteem**:
The physical changes and improvements in strength and functional ability that come with strength training can have a powerful impact on your mental well-being, boosting self-confidence and self-esteem.

Upper Body Exercises

Now that you understand the importance of strength training, it's time to dive into the specific exercises that target and strengthen the muscles of the upper body. These exercises can be performed using various resistance modalities, including free weights, resistance machines, or your own body weight.

1.   **Push-ups**:

One of the most fundamental and effective upper body exercises, push-ups target the chest, shoulders, and triceps muscles. Start in a high plank position with your hands shoulder-width apart, and lower your body until your chest nearly touches the ground, then push back up to the starting position.

Variations: Incline push-ups, decline push-ups, diamond push-ups, and push-up variations using resistance bands or suspension trainers.

2. **Pull-ups/Lat Pull-downs**:

These exercises primarily target the latissimus dorsi (lats) and biceps muscles in the back and arms. For pull-ups, grip an overhead bar with an overhand grip and pull your body up until your chin is above the bar. For lat pull-downs, sit at a pull-down machine and pull the bar down towards your chest, keeping your torso stationary.

Variations: Assisted pull-ups, negatives, and various grip widths for pull-ups; different attachments (straight bar, V-bar, etc.) for lat pull-downs.

3. Bicep Curls:

This exercise targets the biceps brachii, the muscle responsible for flexing the elbow. Stand with your feet shoulder-width apart, holding a dumbbell in each hand with an underhand grip. Keeping your elbows tucked in, curl the weights up towards your shoulders, pause, and then lower them back down in a controlled motion.

Variations: Hammer curls, preacher curls, concentration curls, and using resistance bands or cables for bicep curls.

4. Tricep Extensions:

The triceps brachii, located on the back of the upper arm, is responsible for extending the elbow. For tricep extensions, hold a dumbbell overhead with both hands and lower the weight behind your head, keeping your upper arms stationary. Extend your arms back to the starting position.

Variations: Tricep dips, cable push-downs, and using resistance bands or a straight bar for overhead extensions.

5. **Shoulder Presses**:

This exercise targets the deltoid muscles in the shoulders as well as the triceps. Stand with your feet shoulder-width apart, holding a dumbbell or barbell at shoulder height with an overhand grip. Press the weight directly overhead, pause, and then lower it back to the starting position in a controlled motion.

Variations: Seated dumbbell presses, Arnold presses, and using resistance bands or cables for shoulder presses.

6. **Rows:**

Rowing exercises target the back muscles, including the lats, rhomboids, and biceps. For dumbbell rows, place your left knee and hand on a flat bench, and grip a dumbbell with your right hand. Pull the weight towards your torso, squeezing your back muscles, then lower it back down in a controlled motion. Repeat on the opposite side.

Variations: Seated cable rows, barbell rows, T-bar rows, and using resistance bands for rowing movements.

Tips for Proper Form and Technique

While strength training can yield numerous benefits, it's crucial to prioritize proper form and technique to prevent injuries and maximize the effectiveness of your workouts. Here are some tips to keep in mind:

1. **Warm-up and Cool-down:**

Always begin your strength training sessions with a proper warm-up to prepare your muscles for the upcoming stress and reduce the risk of injury. End your workout with a cool-down and stretching routine to promote recovery and prevent muscle soreness.

2. **Breathing**:

Proper breathing is essential during strength training exercises. Exhale during the concentric (lifting) phase of the movement and inhale during the eccentric (lowering) phase. This can help stabilize your core and maintain proper form.

3. **Controlled Movements**:

Avoid jerky or explosive movements, as these can increase the risk of injury and diminish the effectiveness of the exercise. Focus on controlled, deliberate motions throughout the full range of motion.

4. **Engage Your Core**:

Engage your core muscles by bracing your abdominal region during each exercise. This will help provide stability and support, preventing excessive arching or rounding of the spine.

5. **Gradually Increase Resistance**:

As you become stronger, gradually increase the resistance (weight, bands, etc.) to continue challenging your muscles and promoting growth. However, prioritize proper form over adding weight too quickly.

6. **Listen to Your Body**:

If you experience sharp pain or discomfort during an exercise, stop immediately and reassess your form or consider modifying the movement. Pushing through pain can lead to injury and setbacks in your progress.

7. **Rest and Recovery**:

Allow for adequate rest and recovery between strength training sessions, as this is when muscle growth and repair occur. Aim for at least one to two days of rest between working the same muscle groups.

8. **Seek Guidance:**

If you're new to strength training or unsure about proper form and technique, consider working with a certified personal trainer or attending a beginner's strength training class. Proper guidance can help ensure you're performing exercises correctly and safely.

By incorporating upper body strength training into your routine, you'll not only develop stronger, more defined muscles but also experience a host of additional benefits, including improved bone density, enhanced functional strength, and a boosted metabolism. Remember to prioritize proper form, gradually increase resistance, and listen to your body to ensure a safe and effective strength training journey.

CHAPTER 5

LOWER BODY STRENGTH TRAINING

As you embark on your fitness journey, it's essential to recognize the significance of a well-rounded strength training routine that encompasses both the upper and lower body. While upper body exercises are crucial for building strength and definition in the arms, chest, and back, lower body training is equally important for developing functional strength, improving balance and stability, and enhancing overall athletic performance.

In this chapter, we'll delve into the world of lower body strength training, exploring the numerous benefits it offers and providing you with a comprehensive guide to effective exercises that target the major muscle groups of the legs and core. We'll also emphasize the importance of proper form and technique, as well as the vital role of core strength in maximizing the effectiveness of your lower body workouts.

The Benefits of Lower Body Strength Training

Incorporating lower body strength training into your fitness routine can yield a multitude of benefits that extend far beyond the aesthetic appeal of toned and sculpted legs. Here are some of the most significant advantages:

1. **Increased Functional Strength and Mobility**: Strong and well-developed leg muscles are essential for everyday activities such as walking, climbing stairs, and carrying heavy loads. Lower body strength training can improve your functional strength and mobility, making it easier to perform these tasks with greater ease and efficiency.

2. **Improved Balance and Stability**:

Many lower body exercises, particularly those that involve single-leg movements or dynamic movements like lunges, challenge your balance and stability. By training these skills, you can reduce the risk of falls and injuries, while also enhancing your overall coordination and agility.

3. **Enhanced Athletic Performance:**

Whether you're an avid athlete or simply enjoy recreational sports and activities, lower body strength is a crucial component of athletic performance. Exercises like squats, deadlifts, and plyometrics can improve power, speed, and explosiveness, allowing you to perform better in a wide range of sports and physical endeavors.

4. **Increased Bone Density:**

Weight-bearing exercises that involve the lower body can stimulate the development of new bone tissue, leading to increased bone density and reduced risk of osteoporosis and fractures as you age.

5. **Elevated Metabolism and Fat Loss:**

Lower body exercises engage large muscle groups, such as the quadriceps, hamstrings, and glutes, which can result in a higher caloric expenditure during and after your workout. This elevated metabolism can contribute to increased fat loss and overall weight management.

6. **Improved Posture and Spinal Alignment:**

Strong core and lower body muscles play a vital role in maintaining proper posture and spinal alignment. By strengthening these areas, you can alleviate or prevent issues such as lower back pain, muscle imbalances, and poor posture.

Lower Body Exercises

Now that you understand the numerous benefits of lower body strength training, it's time to explore some of the most effective exercises that target the major muscle groups of the legs and core.

1. **Squats:**

Widely regarded as the king of lower body exercises, squats are a compound movement that engages multiple muscle groups, including the quadriceps, hamstrings, glutes, and core. Start with your feet shoulder-width apart, keeping your chest up and your weight in your heels. Bend your knees and hips, lowering your body as if you're sitting back into a chair, then press through your heels to return to the starting position.

Variations: Back squats, front squats, goblet squats, split squats, and squat jumps.

2. **Lunges:**

Lunges are a unilateral exercise that targets the quadriceps, hamstrings, and glutes of one leg at a time, while also challenging your balance and stability. Step forward with one leg, lowering your body until both knees form 90-degree angles, then push back to the starting position and repeat on the opposite side.

Variations: Reverse lunges, lateral lunges, curtsy lunges, and walking lunges.

3. **Deadlifts**:

Deadlifts are a compound exercise that targets the hamstrings, glutes, and lower back muscles, as well as engaging the core for stability. Start with your feet hip-width apart, hinge at the hips, and bend your knees to grip the barbell or dumbbells on the floor. Keeping your back flat, drive through your heels to stand upright, lifting the weight off the ground.

Variations: Sumo deadlifts, Romanian deadlifts, and single-leg deadlifts.

4. **Leg Presses**:

The leg press machine allows you to target the quadriceps, hamstrings, and glutes through a controlled, seated movement. Sit with your back against the pad, place your feet on the platform, and push the weight away from you by extending your legs. Control the weight on the way back, and repeat.

Variations: Narrow or wide stance, single-leg presses, and elevated or declined foot positioning.

5. **Calf Raises**:

Calf raises target the gastrocnemius and soleus muscles in the calves, which are often neglected in many workout routines. Stand with your feet shoulder-width apart, and raise up onto your toes, lifting your heels off the ground. Pause at the top, then lower back down in a controlled motion.

Variations: Seated calf raises, donkey calf raises, and calf raises with added weight or resistance bands.

6. **Glute Bridges**:

Glute bridges are an excellent exercise for targeting the gluteal muscles, as well as the hamstrings and lower back. Lie on your back with your knees bent and feet flat on the floor. Press through your heels to raise your hips off the ground, forming a straight line from your knees to your shoulders. Squeeze your glutes at the top, then lower back down.

Variations: Single-leg glute bridges, glute bridges with resistance bands or weight plates, and hip thrusts.

Tips for Proper Form and Technique

While these exercises can effectively target and strengthen the muscles of the lower body, it's crucial to prioritize proper form and technique to maximize the benefits and prevent injuries. Here are some tips to keep in mind:

1. **Warm-up and Cool-down**:

Always begin your lower body strength training sessions
with a proper warm-up to prepare your muscles for the
upcoming stress and reduce the risk of injury. End your
workout with a cool-down and stretching routine to
promote recovery and prevent muscle soreness.

2. **Engage Your Core**:

During lower body exercises, it's essential to engage
your core muscles by bracing your abdominal region.
This will help provide stability and support, preventing
excessive arching or rounding of the spine.

3. **Maintain Proper Alignment**:

Pay close attention to your body alignment throughout
each exercise. Keep your chest up, shoulders back, and
avoid excessive arching or rounding of the lower back.

4. **Breathe Properly**:

Proper breathing is crucial during strength training exercises. Exhale during the concentric (lifting) phase of the movement and inhale during the eccentric (lowering) phase. This can help stabilize your core and maintain proper form.

5.   Control the Movement:

Avoid jerky or explosive movements, as these can increase the risk of injury and diminish the effectiveness of the exercise. Focus on controlled, deliberate motions throughout the full range of motion.

6.   Gradually Increase Resistance:

As you become stronger, gradually increase the resistance (weight, bands, etc.) to continue challenging your muscles and promoting growth. However, prioritize proper form over adding weight too quickly.

7.   Listen to Your Body:

If you experience sharp pain or discomfort during an exercise, stop immediately and reassess your form or consider modifying the movement. Pushing through pain can lead to injury and setbacks in your progress.

8. **Seek Guidance**:

If you're new to strength training or unsure about proper form and technique, consider working with a certified personal trainer or attending a beginner's strength training class. Proper guidance can help ensure you're performing exercises correctly and safely.

The Importance of Core Strength

While lower body strength training primarily targets the muscles of the legs, it's essential to recognize the vital role that core strength plays in maximizing the effectiveness and safety of these exercises. Your core muscles, which include the abdominal muscles, obliques, and lower back muscles, act as a stabilizing force during compound movements like squats, lunges, and deadlifts.

A strong and engaged core helps maintain proper spinal alignment, reduces the risk of injury, and allows you to generate more power and force from your lower body. Many lower body exercises, such as the deadlift and squat, inherently challenge and strengthen the core muscles, but it's also beneficial to incorporate dedicated core exercises into your routine.

Examples of effective core exercises include:
1. Planks (front, side, and reverse)
2. Russian Twists
3. Dead Bugs
4. Hollow Body Holds
5. Pallof Presses
6. Cable Chops/Lifts
7. Hanging Leg Raises
8. Ab Wheel Rollouts

By consistently training your core muscles in conjunction with your lower body exercises, you'll not only enhance the effectiveness of your workouts but also improve your overall strength, stability, and posture.

Remember, lower body strength training is a crucial component of a well-rounded fitness routine. By incorporating exercises like squats, lunges, deadlifts, and calf raises into your regimen, you'll not only develop powerful and sculpted legs but also reap the numerous benefits of improved functional strength, balance, athletic performance, and overall physical capability.

As with any strength training program, it's essential to prioritize proper form and technique, engage your core muscles, and gradually increase resistance to continue challenging your body and promoting growth. With dedication, patience, and a commitment to safe and effective training, you'll be well on your way to unlocking the full potential of your lower body strength

and taking your fitness journey to new heights.

CHAPTER 6

CORE STRENGTHENING EXERCISES

At the heart of every powerful, efficient, and injury-free movement lies a strong and stable core. The core muscles, often referred to as the body's powerhouse, play a crucial role in maintaining proper posture, enhancing balance, and facilitating the transfer of force throughout the kinetic chain. In this chapter, we'll delve into the importance of core strength, explore a variety of effective core exercises, and provide practical tips for seamlessly incorporating these essential movements into your routine.

The Importance of Core Strength

Before we dive into the exercises, it's essential to understand why cultivating core strength should be a priority in your fitness journey. A strong and stable core not only enhances your overall performance but also contributes to numerous benefits, including:

1. **Improved Posture:**

The core muscles, including the abdominals, lower back muscles, and the muscles surrounding the hips and pelvis, play a crucial role in maintaining proper spinal alignment and upright posture. By strengthening these muscles, you'll be better equipped to support the weight of your upper body, reducing strain on the back and minimizing the risk of slouching or developing poor posture habits.

2. **Enhanced Balance and Stability:**

The core acts as a stabilizing force, allowing for efficient transfer of power from your lower body to your upper body, and vice versa. A strong core enables better balance and stability during various movements, such as squats, lunges, and any exercise that challenges your equilibrium. This improved stability not only enhances your performance but also reduces the risk of falls and injuries.

3. Increased Functional Strength:

Strong core muscles are essential for everyday activities, such as lifting, carrying, and even sitting or standing for prolonged periods. By strengthening your core, you'll improve your overall functional strength, making daily tasks easier and reducing the risk of injury from simple movements.

4. Reduced Risk of Back Pain:

Weak or imbalanced core muscles can contribute to lower back pain, as they fail to provide adequate support and stability to the spine. By targeting and strengthening the core muscles, you can alleviate existing back pain and prevent future issues, leading to improved overall comfort and mobility.

5. Enhanced Athletic Performance:

For athletes and fitness enthusiasts alike, a strong core is the foundation for generating power, transferring force efficiently, and maintaining proper form during various sports and activities. Whether you're a runner, cyclist, weightlifter, or participate in any other physical pursuit, a robust core can significantly improve your performance and reduce the risk of injury.

The Core Muscles: Anatomy and Function

Before we dive into specific exercises, it's essential to understand the core muscles and their primary functions. The core is a complex system made up of several muscle groups, including:

1. **Rectus Abdominis:**

Often referred to as the "six-pack" muscles, the rectus abdominis runs vertically along the front of the abdomen. Its primary function is flexing the spine, such as during sit-ups or crunches.

2. **Obliques**:

The internal and external oblique muscles are located on the sides of the abdomen and are responsible for rotating and laterally flexing the trunk.

3. **Transverse Abdominis**:

The deepest abdominal muscle, the transverse abdominis, wraps around the midsection like a corset. Its primary function is stabilizing the spine and providing intra-abdominal pressure.

4. **Erector Spinae**:

The erector spinae is a group of muscles that run along the length of the spine, from the base of the skull to the pelvis. These muscles are responsible for extending and laterally flexing the spine.

5. **Multifidus**:

The multifidus muscles are small, deep muscles that run parallel to the erector spinae. They play a crucial role in stabilizing the individual vertebrae of the spine.

6. **Quadratus Lumborum**:

The quadratus lumborum muscles are located on either side of the lower back and are responsible for laterally flexing and stabilizing the spine.

7. Hip Muscles:

The hip muscles, including the gluteus maximus, gluteus medius, and hip flexors, play a vital role in core stability and are essential for generating power and maintaining proper form during various movements.

By understanding the anatomy and function of these core muscles, you'll be better equipped to target and strengthen them effectively, leading to improved overall stability, performance, and injury prevention.

Effective Core Exercises

Now that we've explored the importance of core strength and the muscles involved, let's dive into a variety of effective core exercises that can be incorporated into your routine. Remember, when performing these exercises, it's crucial to maintain proper form and engage the core muscles throughout the movement.

1. Planks:

The plank is a foundational core exercise that engages multiple muscle groups, including the rectus abdominis, obliques, and erector spinae. Start in a push-up position, supporting your weight on your forearms and toes. Engage your core by drawing your navel inward, and maintain a straight line from your head to your heels. Hold this position for as long as possible, aiming for a minimum of 30 seconds to start.

Variations:

- Side Planks: Shift your weight onto one forearm, stacking your feet on top of each other, and raise your hips off the ground, forming a straight line from your ankles to your shoulders.

- Plank Jacks: From a standard plank position, jump your feet out to the sides and back together, mimicking a jumping jack motion.

- Plank Shoulder Taps: From a standard plank position, lift one hand off the ground and tap the opposite shoulder, alternating sides.

2. Dead Bugs:

The dead bug exercise is an excellent choice for targeting the deep core muscles, particularly the transverse abdominis. Begin by lying on your back with your arms extended towards the ceiling and your legs raised, forming a 90-degree angle with your torso. Engage your core by drawing your navel inward. Slowly extend one leg out while reaching the opposite arm back, keeping your lower back pressed into the ground.

Alternate sides, focusing on controlled movements and maintaining core engagement.

3. Russian Twists:

The Russian twist is a dynamic exercise that targets the obliques and challenges core stability. Sit on the floor with your knees bent and feet flat on the ground. Lean back slightly, engaging your core, and lift your feet off the floor, balancing on your sit bones. With your arms extended in front of you, twist your torso to the right, then to the left, touching the ground on each side if possible. Keep your movements controlled and your core engaged throughout the exercise.

4. Hollow Body Holds:

The hollow body hold is an advanced core exercise that targets multiple muscle groups simultaneously. Begin by lying on your back with your arms extended overhead and your legs straight out in front of you. Engage your core by pressing your lower back into the ground and raising your arms, legs, and shoulder blades off the floor. Hold this position, maintaining tension throughout your entire body, for as long as possible.

5. Leg Raises:

Leg raises are an effective exercise for targeting the lower abdominals and hip flexors. Start by lying on your back with your legs extended and your hands placed beside you for support. Keeping your legs straight, slowly raise them up towards the ceiling, focusing on using your core muscles to lift them. Once you reach the highest point you can comfortably achieve, slowly lower your legs back down, maintaining control throughout the movement.

Variations:

- Reverse Crunches: From the leg raise position, use your core muscles to lift your hips off the ground, bringing your knees towards your chest.

- Flutter Kicks: While lying on your back, raise your legs a few inches off the ground and perform small, controlled kicks, alternating between each leg.

6. Bird Dogs:

The bird dog exercise is a fantastic way to challenge core stability while incorporating movement and coordination. Start on your hands and knees, with your hands directly under your shoulders and your knees under your hips. Engage your core by drawing your navel inward. Simultaneously extend one arm and the opposite leg, creating a straight line from your fingertips to your toes. Hold for a few seconds, then switch sides, alternating between each arm and leg.

7. Mountain Climbers:

Mountain climbers are a dynamic exercise that incorporates core stability with cardiovascular conditioning. Start in a high plank position, with your hands directly under your shoulders. Engage your core and bring one knee towards your chest, then quickly switch and bring the other knee in, mimicking a climbing motion. Continue alternating legs, maintaining a steady pace and keeping your core engaged throughout the movement.

Tips for Incorporating Core Exercises into Your Routine

Now that you've explored a variety of effective core exercises, it's time to discuss how to seamlessly integrate them into your workout routine. Here are some practical tips:

1. Warm-up and Cool-down:

Before diving into your core routine, ensure you properly warm up your body with light cardio and dynamic stretches. This will prepare your muscles for the upcoming work and reduce the risk of injury. Similarly, end your core workout with a cool-down routine, such as gentle stretches or foam rolling, to facilitate recovery and prevent soreness.

2. Dedicated Core Days:

Consider dedicating specific days in your weekly routine to focused core training. This approach allows you to target your core muscles with greater intensity and variety, without being limited by fatigue from other exercises.

3. Circuit Training:

Incorporate core exercises into your existing strength training or circuit routines. You can strategically place core movements between sets of other exercises, creating a well-rounded and efficient workout.

4. Finishers:

After completing your primary workout, add a core "finisher" at the end. This could be a challenging plank variation, a set of Russian twists, or a combination of core exercises to really challenge and fatigue your midsection.

5. Active Rest:

During rest periods between sets or exercises, engage your core with isometric holds or low-intensity core movements. This approach keeps your core engaged throughout the entire workout, maximizing the overall training stimulus.

6. Progression and Variety:

As with any exercise routine, it's essential to progressively increase the difficulty and introduce variety to avoid plateaus and continue challenging your core muscles. This could involve adding resistance (e.g., weight plates or medicine balls), increasing the duration of holds, or exploring new variations of exercises.

7. Mind-Muscle Connection:

Throughout your core exercises, maintain a strong mind-muscle connection by consciously engaging and squeezing your core muscles. This mental focus will not only enhance the effectiveness of the exercises but also improve your overall body awareness and control.

8. Balanced Approach:

While core training is crucial, it's essential to maintain a balanced approach and incorporate exercises that target all major muscle groups. A well-rounded routine that includes strength training, cardiovascular exercise, and flexibility work will ensure overall fitness and prevent muscle imbalances.

Remember, consistency and proper form are key when it comes to core training. Always prioritize quality over quantity, and listen to your body's signals to avoid overtraining or injury. With dedication and patience, you'll soon experience the transformative power of a strong, stable core - improved posture, enhanced balance, increased functional strength, and a reduced risk of back pain.

Embrace the challenge of core strengthening exercises, and watch as your fitness journey reaches new heights of performance, confidence, and overall well-being. A strong core is the foundation upon which all other physical pursuits are built, so make it a priority, and reap the countless benefits that come with a powerful, resilient midsection.

CHAPTER 7

FLEXIBILITY AND MOBILITY EXERCISES

In the pursuit of a well-rounded and effective fitness routine, it's easy to overlook the importance of flexibility and mobility exercises. While many individuals focus their efforts on cardiovascular endurance and strength training, neglecting this vital component can have far-reaching consequences on overall physical function, performance, and injury prevention.

Flexibility and mobility are often used interchangeably, but they represent distinct yet interconnected aspects of physical fitness. In this chapter, we'll explore the nuances of each, delve into their numerous benefits, and provide you with a comprehensive guide to effective flexibility and mobility exercises, equipping you with the knowledge and tools to seamlessly incorporate these essential practices into your routine.

Flexibility refers to the ability of a muscle or group of muscles to lengthen and extend through their full range of motion. It's a critical component of physical fitness that allows for unrestricted movement and can help prevent injuries resulting from excessive muscle tightness or restricted joint mobility.

Mobility, on the other hand, is the ability to move a joint or series of joints through their full range of motion without restriction. This encompasses not only the flexibility of the muscles surrounding the joint but also the joint structure itself, including the bones, ligaments, and tendons.

While flexibility and mobility are closely related, it's possible to have one without the other. For example, an individual may have flexible muscles but limited joint mobility due to structural restrictions, or vice versa.

Achieving optimal physical function and minimizing the risk of injury requires addressing both flexibility and mobility through targeted exercises and stretching routines.

The Importance of Flexibility and Mobility

Incorporating flexibility and mobility exercises into your fitness routine can yield numerous benefits that extend far beyond the physical realm. Here are some of the most significant advantages:

1. **Improved Range of Motion**:

By consistently working on flexibility and mobility, you can increase your range of motion, allowing for greater freedom of movement and improved overall physical function. This can enhance your performance in various activities, from sports and recreational pursuits to daily tasks like bending, reaching, and lifting.

2. **Injury Prevention**:

Tight muscles and limited joint mobility can increase the risk of strains, sprains, and other injuries, particularly during physical activity. By improving flexibility and mobility, you can reduce the likelihood of these injuries and protect your body from the stresses of exercise and daily movements.

3.   Enhanced Athletic Performance:

For athletes and active individuals, optimal flexibility and mobility can translate into improved power, speed, and overall performance. Increased range of motion allows for more efficient and explosive movements, while reduced muscle tightness can improve technique and form.

4.   Improved Posture:

Muscle imbalances and tightness can contribute to poor posture, leading to discomfort, pain, and potential long-term issues like muscle strains and joint dysfunction. By addressing flexibility and mobility, you can help restore proper alignment and improve your overall posture.

5. **Reduced Muscle Soreness**:

Regular stretching and mobility exercises can help alleviate muscle soreness and promote recovery after intense workouts or physical activity. This can allow you to maintain consistency in your training and continue making progress towards your fitness goals.

6. **Increased Mindfulness and Relaxation**:

Many flexibility and mobility exercises, such as yoga and static stretching, encourage mindfulness and deep breathing, which can promote relaxation and reduce stress levels. This can have a positive impact on both physical and mental well-being.

Flexibility Exercises

Now that you understand the significance of flexibility and mobility, let's explore some effective exercises to improve these important components of physical fitness.

1. **Hamstring Stretches**:

- Seated Forward Fold: Sit on the floor with your legs extended in front of you. Reach forward, keeping your back straight, and gently fold over your legs, reaching toward your toes.

- Standing Hamstring Stretch: Stand with one leg elevated on a bench or chair. Keeping your back straight, hinge forward at the hips, reaching your hands toward your elevated foot.

2. **Hip Flexor Stretches**:

- Kneeling Hip Flexor Stretch: Kneel on one knee, with your other leg extended in front of you, foot flat on the floor. Gently lean your hips forward, keeping your upper body upright, to feel the stretch in the front of your hip.

-   Butterfly Stretch: Sit on the floor with the soles of your feet together, knees bent outward. Gently press down on your knees with your elbows to deepen the stretch in your inner thighs and groin area.

3. **Quadriceps Stretches**:

-   Standing Quad Stretch: Stand with one hand on a wall for balance. Bend one knee and grab your ankle or foot, gently pulling your heel toward your glutes.

-   Kneeling Quad Stretch: Kneel on one knee, with your other leg extended in front of you. Keeping your upper body upright, lean back, feeling the stretch in the front of your thigh.

4. **Calf Stretches**:

-   Wall Calf Stretch: Stand facing a wall, with your hands against the wall at shoulder height. Step back with one leg, keeping your heel on the ground, and lean forward to feel the stretch in your calf.

- Runner's Calf Stretch: In a split stance, with one leg forward and one leg back, bend your front knee and lean forward, keeping your back heel on the ground.

5. **Upper Body Stretches**:

- Overhead Triceps Stretch: Raise one arm overhead and bend your elbow, reaching your hand down between your shoulder blades. Use your other hand to gently pull the stretching arm closer to your head.

- Chest Stretch: Stand in a doorway or corner, with your arms extended and hands at shoulder height on the walls or doorframe. Step forward with one leg, feeling the stretch across your chest and shoulders.

Mobility Exercises

While flexibility exercises focus on lengthening and stretching specific muscle groups, mobility exercises target the joints and their surrounding structures, promoting unrestricted movement and range of motion.

1. **Arm Circles:**

Stand with your feet shoulder-width apart and extend your arms out to the sides, parallel to the ground. Make small, controlled circles with your arms, gradually increasing the size of the circles. Reverse the direction and repeat.

2. **Hip Circles:**

Stand with your feet shoulder-width apart and place your hands on your hips. Keeping your upper body stable, make small circles with your hips, gradually increasing the size of the circles. Reverse the direction and repeat.

3. **Ankle Mobility:**

Sit or stand with one foot elevated on a chair or bench. Using your hands, gently rotate your ankle in a circular motion, moving through the full range of motion. Repeat on the other side.

4. **Thoracic Spine Rotation**:

Lie on your side with your knees bent and your hips and shoulders stacked. Keeping your hips and knees together, rotate your upper body and reach your arm across your body, feeling a stretch in your mid-back and shoulder area. Repeat on the other side.

5. **Inchworm**:

Start in a standing position, and hinge forward at the hips to place your hands on the floor, keeping your legs straight. Walk your hands out, one at a time, until you're in a plank position. Hold for a moment, then walk your feet back towards your hands, returning to the standing position.

Now that you have a solid understanding of flexibility and mobility exercises, it's time to learn how to effectively incorporate them into your fitness routine:

1. **Warm-up and Cool-down**:

Always include flexibility and mobility exercises in your warm-up and cool-down routines. Start your workout sessions with dynamic stretches and mobility drills to prepare your body for the upcoming physical demands, and end with static stretches to promote recovery and prevent muscle soreness.

2. **Dedicate Specific Training Sessions**:

In addition to incorporating flexibility and mobility exercises into your warm-up and cool-down routines, consider dedicating specific training sessions to focus solely on these components. This can be especially beneficial for individuals with significant tightness or mobility restrictions.

3. **Tailor Your Routine**:

Assess your individual needs and tailor your flexibility and mobility routine accordingly. If you have areas of particular tightness or limited range of motion, prioritize exercises that target those specific muscle groups or joints.

4. **Consistency is Key**:

As with any aspect of physical fitness, consistency is crucial for achieving and maintaining optimal flexibility and mobility. Aim to incorporate these exercises into your routine at least two to three times per week, or even daily for those with significant restrictions.

5. **Breathe Deeply**:

During static stretches and mobility exercises, focus on deep, controlled breathing. This can help you relax into the stretch, maximize its effectiveness, and promote a sense of mindfulness and relaxation.

6. **Gradually Increase Intensity**:

As with any form of exercise, it's important to gradually increase the intensity and duration of your flexibility and mobility routine. Avoid pushing too hard too soon, as this can increase the risk of injury and potentially cause setbacks in your progress.

7. **Listen to Your Body**:

Pay attention to how your body feels during and after your flexibility and mobility exercises. If you experience sharp pain or discomfort, ease off or stop the exercise altogether. Flexibility and mobility should be achieved through gentle, controlled movements, not forced.

8. **Incorporate Recovery Techniques**:

Complement your flexibility and mobility routine with other recovery techniques, such as foam rolling, self-myofascial release, and gentle active recovery exercises. These can help promote muscle relaxation, alleviate soreness, and further improve overall mobility.

9. Stay Hydrated:

Proper hydration is essential for optimal physical performance, including flexibility and mobility exercises. Make sure to drink plenty of water before, during, and after your routine to support muscle function and recovery.

10. Consider Professional Guidance:

If you're new to flexibility and mobility exercises or have specific concerns or limitations, consider seeking guidance from a qualified professional, such as a certified personal trainer, physical therapist, or yoga instructor. They can provide personalized advice, ensure proper form and technique, and help you develop a safe and effective routine.

By prioritizing flexibility and mobility exercises and incorporating them into your overall fitness routine, you'll not only improve your range of motion and reduce the risk of injury but also enhance your overall physical performance, posture, and quality of life. Remember, flexibility and mobility are essential components of a well-rounded fitness program and should be given the attention they deserve.

CHAPTER 8

HIGH-INTENSITY INTERVAL TRAINING (HIIT)

In the ever-evolving landscape of fitness, one training method has emerged as a powerful and efficient way to challenge your body, boost your cardiovascular health, and ignite your metabolism: High-Intensity Interval Training, or HIIT. This innovative approach to exercise has gained widespread popularity among fitness enthusiasts, athletes, and busy individuals alike, offering a time-efficient way to maximize results while keeping workouts engaging and dynamic.

In this chapter, we'll delve into the science behind HIIT, explore its numerous benefits, and provide you with a comprehensive guide to implementing this training style into your routine. From heart-pumping exercises to practical tips for beginners, this section will equip you with the knowledge and tools to harness the transformative power of HIIT and take your fitness journey to new heights.

Understanding High-Intensity Interval Training

HIIT is a form of cardiovascular exercise that alternates brief periods of intense anaerobic effort with periods of lower-intensity recovery. Unlike traditional steady-state cardio, which involves maintaining a consistent pace or intensity throughout the workout, HIIT pushes your body to its limits during the high-intensity intervals, followed by periods of active recovery.

The intense bursts of effort during HIIT workouts can range from 20 seconds to several minutes, depending on the specific protocol and your fitness level. These intense intervals are then followed by recovery periods that are typically equal to or slightly longer than the work intervals, allowing your body to partially recover before the next intense effort.

The science behind HIIT lies in its ability to challenge your body's various energy systems and elicit a unique physiological response. During the high-intensity intervals, your body primarily relies on anaerobic metabolism, which breaks down stored glycogen (carbohydrates) for energy without the presence of oxygen. This process is inherently intense and can't be sustained for prolonged periods, hence the need for recovery intervals.

The Benefits of High-Intensity Interval Training

HIIT has gained widespread popularity for a reason – it offers a multitude of benefits that extend far beyond traditional steady-state cardio workouts. Here are some of the most notable advantages of incorporating HIIT into your fitness routine:

1. **Improved Cardiovascular Health:**

HIIT workouts effectively challenge and improve your cardiovascular system by forcing your heart to work harder during the high-intensity intervals. This increased demand on your heart and lungs can lead to improved oxygen uptake, increased stroke volume (the amount of blood pumped per beat), and overall cardiovascular endurance.

2. **Increased Calorie Burn and Fat Loss:**

One of the most attractive benefits of HIIT is its ability to burn a significant number of calories in a relatively short amount of time. The intense nature of the intervals, combined with the increased metabolic demand during the recovery phases, can lead to a higher overall calorie burn compared to steady-state cardio workouts of the same duration.

3. **Boosted Metabolism:**

HIIT workouts have been shown to have a significant impact on your metabolism, even after the workout is over. This phenomenon, known as the "afterburn effect" or excess post-exercise oxygen consumption (EPOC), refers to the increased calorie burn and elevated metabolic rate that can last for several hours after a HIIT session.

4. **Time Efficiency**:

In our fast-paced, modern lives, finding the time to dedicate to lengthy workout sessions can be a challenge. HIIT workouts offer a time-efficient solution, allowing you to achieve significant fitness benefits in a relatively short amount of time, often ranging from 20 to 45 minutes.

5. **Increased Muscular Endurance and Strength**:

While HIIT is primarily considered a cardiovascular training method, many HIIT workouts incorporate resistance exercises or bodyweight movements like push-ups, squats, and burpees. These exercises not only challenge your cardiovascular system but also contribute to increased muscular endurance and strength.

6. **Improved Insulin Sensitivity**:

Regular HIIT training has been linked to improved insulin sensitivity, which can help regulate blood sugar levels and reduce the risk of developing type 2 diabetes. By challenging your body's energy systems, HIIT can enhance your cells' ability to utilize glucose effectively, leading to better metabolic health.

HIIT Workout Examples

Now that you understand the principles and benefits of HIIT, it's time to explore some practical examples of HIIT workouts you can incorporate into your routine. Remember, the key to an effective HIIT session is to push yourself to your maximum effort during the intense intervals while allowing for sufficient recovery periods.

1. **Tabata Protocol**:

The Tabata protocol is a classic HIIT workout that consists of 20 seconds of maximum effort followed by 10 seconds of rest, repeated for a total of 8 rounds (4 minutes). This intense protocol can be performed with various exercises, such as burpees, squat jumps, or high knees.

2. **Sprint Intervals**:

Sprint intervals are a simple yet challenging HIIT workout that can be performed on a treadmill, track, or even outdoors. After a warm-up, alternate between periods of all-out sprinting (e.g., 30 seconds) and periods of active recovery (e.g., 60 seconds of walking or jogging).

3. **Bodyweight Circuit**:

Create a circuit of bodyweight exercises like push-ups, squats, lunges, and mountain climbers, and perform each exercise for a set amount of time (e.g., 30 seconds) with minimal rest between exercises. Complete the circuit multiple times for a full-body HIIT workout.

4. **Battle Ropes**:

Battle ropes are a versatile and intense HIIT tool that can be used for various exercises, such as waves, slams, and alternating arm movements. Perform intervals of intense rope work followed by periods of rest or active recovery.

5. **Kettlebell Swings**:

Kettlebell swings are a highly effective HIIT exercise that targets multiple muscle groups while providing a cardiovascular challenge. Alternate between periods of intense swinging (e.g., 30 seconds) and periods of rest or active recovery.

6. **Cycling Sprints**:

If you have access to a stationary bike or spin bike, incorporate cycling sprints into your HIIT routine. After a warm-up, alternate between periods of all-out sprinting (e.g., 30 seconds) and periods of active recovery (e.g., 60 seconds of easy pedaling).

While HIIT workouts can be incredibly effective, it's important to approach them with caution and follow some practical guidelines to ensure safety and maximize results:

1. **Start Slowly:**

If you're new to HIIT, it's essential to start slowly and gradually increase the intensity and duration of your workouts. Begin with shorter intervals (e.g., 20 seconds) and longer recovery periods (e.g., 40 seconds), and gradually increase the work-to-rest ratio as you become more conditioned.

2. **Warm-up Properly:**

HIIT workouts place significant demands on your body, so it's crucial to warm up properly before each session. A dynamic warm-up that includes movements like high knees, butt kicks, and arm swings can help prepare your muscles and cardiovascular system for the intense work ahead.

3. **Listen to Your Body:**

HIIT workouts are designed to push you to your limits, but it's important to listen to your body and avoid pushing too hard, too soon. If you feel dizzy, lightheaded, or experience any sharp pain, stop the workout immediately and seek medical attention if necessary.

4. **Incorporate Recovery Days:**

While HIIT can be an effective training tool, it's important to avoid overtraining and allow your body adequate time to recover between intense sessions. Aim to incorporate HIIT workouts 2-3 times per week, with at least one full day of rest or active recovery in between.

5. **Vary Your Workouts**:

To prevent plateaus and keep your body challenged, it's important to vary your HIIT workouts. Experiment with different exercises, intervals, and intensities to continually push your body out of its comfort zone and promote continuous progress.

6. **Stay Hydrated**:

HIIT workouts can be incredibly demanding and lead to significant fluid loss through sweat. Make sure to stay hydrated by drinking water before, during, and after your HIIT sessions to support optimal performance and recovery.

7. **Consider Your Fitness Level**:

HIIT workouts can be scaled to accommodate various fitness levels, but it's important to be honest about your current capabilities. If you're new to exercise or have any underlying health conditions, it may be beneficial to consult with a certified personal trainer or healthcare professional before starting a HIIT program.

By incorporating HIIT into your fitness routine, you'll not only maximize the effectiveness of your workouts but also experience a renewed sense of motivation and progress. With its time-efficient approach and dynamic workout structure, HIIT takes your fitness journey to new levels, consistently challenging you both physically and mentally.

The variety of HIIT workouts presented in this comprehensive guide allows you to explore a wide range of high-intensity training methods tailored to your preferences and goals. From quick yet intense HIIT circuits designed to push your limits, to creative workout combinations that keep your sessions engaging and inspiring, you'll find a diverse array of tailored HIIT programs.

This unique approach maximizes the impact of each workout experience while ensuring your training remains refreshingly varied, preventing the monotony that can often hinder motivation and progress. By incorporating the dynamic HIIT techniques outlined in this resource, you'll unlock new dimensions of fitness while elevating your journey to new levels of achievement.

HIIT's distinct application of carefully crafted high-intensity intervals seamlessly integrates physical conditioning with an engaging experience, amplifying the comprehensive impact of every workout session. As you explore the tailored HIIT programs presented here, you'll experience a refreshing evolution of training that harmonizes effective physical development with enriching variety, continuously inspiring dedication and progress along your personalized fitness path.

Immersing yourself in the HIIT approach, you'll cultivate a harmonious synergy between efficient training and an engaging fitness experience that continuously elevates your commitment and achievement. This focused application of HIIT techniques will guide you on a uniquely inspiring journey, fostering dedication and refinement through the very essence of each meticulously crafted workout experience.

Moreover, as you embrace this HIIT-centric approach, you'll find that the very intensity and structure of these workout experiences foster a sustained commitment and sense of accomplishment. The focused expression of tailored conditioning, integrated with creatively diverse applications, imbues your entire fitness journey with a cohesive dynamic, enriching your development and inspiring an elevated dedication to progress.

As this comprehensive exploration of HIIT principles shapes an engaging experience that resonates with the very essence of your dedicated fitness journey, you'll transcend conventional boundaries, harmonizing physical aptitude with diverse applications of conditioning, all harmonized by the very nature of this concentrated approach.

In essence, this concentrated progression inherently catalyzes an elevated experience, harnessing the essence of personalized conditioning while simultaneously cultivating refined dedication through the contextual dynamic inherent in the focused paradigm of HIIT.

CHAPTER 9

PROGRESSIVE OVERLOAD AND PROGRESSIVE RESISTANCE

As you embark on your fitness journey, it's essential to understand the principles that govern progress and growth. Consistency and dedication are undoubtedly crucial, but without the proper application of progressive overload and progressive resistance, your efforts may plateau, leaving you feeling stagnant and unfulfilled. In this chapter, we'll delve into the science behind these fundamental concepts, explore their importance in achieving your fitness goals, and provide you with practical tips and strategies to seamlessly incorporate progressive overload and progressive resistance into your workout routine.

Progressive overload is a fundamental principle in exercise science that states that to continually make progress and see results, you must gradually increase the demands placed on your body over time. This principle applies to all aspects of physical fitness, including strength training, cardiovascular exercise, and flexibility.

When you engage in physical activity, your body adapts to the stress imposed upon it. Initially, these adaptations may result in increased strength, endurance, or flexibility. However, if the same level of stress is consistently applied, your body will eventually reach a plateau, and progress will stall. This is where progressive overload comes into play.

By gradually increasing the intensity, volume, or resistance of your workouts, you create a new stimulus that challenges your body to adapt further. This can be achieved through various methods, such as increasing the weight lifted, adding more repetitions or sets, increasing the duration or intensity of cardiovascular exercise, or introducing new exercises or variations.

The Importance of Progressive Overload

Incorporating progressive overload into your workout routine is essential for several reasons:

1. **Continued Muscle Growth and Strength Gains:** When it comes to building muscle and increasing strength, progressive overload is the driving force behind your progress. By gradually increasing the weight or resistance you're working against, you create a stimulus that forces your muscles to adapt and grow stronger.

2. **Improved Cardiovascular Endurance:** Progressive overload is equally important for enhancing cardiovascular endurance. By gradually increasing the intensity, duration, or complexity of your cardio

workouts, you challenge your cardiovascular system to adapt and become more efficient.

3. **Increased Flexibility and Mobility:**

Even flexibility and mobility can benefit from progressive overload. By gradually increasing the range of motion or intensity of your stretching and mobility exercises, you can continue to improve your overall flexibility and functional movement capabilities.

4. **Preventing Plateaus:**

Without progressive overload, your body will eventually adapt to the demands placed upon it, resulting in a plateau where progress stalls. By consistently increasing the challenge, you prevent this plateau and keep your body adapting and improving.

Understanding Progressive Resistance

Progressive resistance is a specific application of progressive overload that focuses on gradually increasing the resistance or weight used during strength training exercises. This principle is particularly important for those seeking to build muscle mass, increase strength, and develop functional power.

When you lift weights or engage in resistance training, your muscles are placed under tension, causing microscopic tears in the muscle fibers. As these fibers repair themselves during the recovery process, they become stronger and slightly larger, leading to muscle growth and increased strength.

However, for this process to continue, you must consistently challenge your muscles with increased resistance or weight. If you continue to lift the same weight or resistance over time, your muscles will eventually adapt, and progress will stall.

The Importance of Progressive Resistance

Incorporating progressive resistance into your strength training routine is crucial for several reasons:

1. **Increased Muscle Growth**:

By progressively increasing the resistance or weight you're lifting, you create a stimulus that forces your muscles to adapt and grow larger to handle the increased demand. This is the primary mechanism by which muscles are built and sculpted.

2. **Improved Strength and Power**:

In addition to muscle growth, progressive resistance also plays a vital role in increasing your overall strength and power. As your muscles adapt to the increased resistance, they become better equipped to generate greater force, leading to improved performance in various physical activities.

3. **Functional Strength Development**:

Progressive resistance training not only builds muscle and strength but also translates to improved functional strength for everyday activities. As you become stronger and more capable of handling heavier loads, tasks like lifting, carrying, and pushing become easier and less taxing on your body.

4. **Metabolic Boost**:

Resistance training, particularly when combined with progressive overload, can have a significant impact on your metabolism. The increased muscle mass resulting from progressive resistance training requires more energy (calories) to maintain, leading to a higher overall metabolic rate and potential fat loss.

Tips for Incorporating Progressive Overload and Progressive Resistance

Now that you understand the importance of progressive overload and progressive resistance, it's time to explore practical strategies for incorporating these principles into your workout routine:

1. **Start Light and Focus on Form**:

Before attempting to increase weight or resistance, it's crucial to master proper form and technique. Start with lighter weights or resistance levels and focus on executing each exercise with good form. This will not only reduce the risk of injury but also ensure that you're engaging the correct muscle groups effectively.

2. **Gradually Increase Weight or Resistance**:

Once you've mastered proper form, you can begin to gradually increase the weight or resistance you're working with. A general guideline is to increase the weight by 5-10% when you can comfortably perform the desired number of repetitions with good form.

3. **Vary Your Rep Ranges:**

Incorporating different rep ranges into your routine can help stimulate muscle growth and strength gains in different ways. Higher rep ranges (12-15 reps) can promote muscular endurance and metabolic stress, while lower rep ranges (4-6 reps) can target maximum strength and power.

4. **Periodize Your Training**:

Periodization involves strategically varying your training variables (intensity, volume, exercise selection, etc.) over time to continually challenge your body and prevent plateaus. This can involve rotating through different rep ranges, adjusting rest periods, or introducing new exercises or training methods.

5. **Track Your Progress**:

Keeping a detailed workout log is essential for monitoring your progress and ensuring that you're consistently increasing the demands placed on your body. Record the weight, reps, sets, and any other relevant details for each exercise, allowing you to accurately track your progress and make informed decisions about when to increase the intensity.

6. **Listen to Your Body**:

While progressive overload and progressive resistance are essential for continued progress, it's equally important to listen to your body and avoid pushing too hard, too soon. If you experience excessive soreness, fatigue, or a decline in performance, it may be a sign that you need to dial back the intensity or take a deload week to allow for recovery.

7. **Incorporate Deload Weeks**:

Deload weeks involve strategically reducing the intensity and volume of your workouts for a short period, typically one week every 4-8 weeks. This temporary reduction in stress allows your body to recover and can help prevent overtraining and plateaus in the long run.

8. **Seek Professional Guidance:**

If you're new to strength training or unsure about how to properly implement progressive overload and progressive resistance, consider seeking guidance from a certified personal trainer or experienced coach. They can help you develop a personalized program and ensure that you're progressing safely and effectively.

By embracing the principles of progressive overload and progressive resistance, you'll unlock the true potential of your fitness journey. These fundamental concepts will not only drive continued progress and prevent plateaus but also foster a mindset of constant growth and improvement. Remember, true transformation occurs when you constantly challenge yourself and push beyond your perceived limits.

CHAPTER 10

WORKOUT ROUTINES FOR DIFFERENT GOALS

As you progress on your fitness journey, it's important to recognize that different goals may require tailored approaches to exercise and training. While the foundational principles of proper form, progressive overload, and balanced programming remain constant, the specific emphasis and structure of your workout routine can vary depending on whether your primary objective is weight loss, muscle gain, improved endurance, or overall functional fitness.

In this chapter, we'll explore workout routines designed to address various fitness goals, providing you with practical examples and actionable strategies to help you create a personalized program that aligns with your specific aspirations. Whether you're seeking to shed excess body fat, build lean muscle mass, enhance your cardiovascular endurance, or simply improve your overall physical capabilities, you'll find a comprehensive guide to help you navigate the path to success.

Weight Loss Workout Routine

If your primary goal is to lose weight and reduce body fat, your workout routine should focus on creating a caloric deficit through a combination of cardiovascular exercise and resistance training. Here's an example of a well-rounded weight loss workout routine:

Day 1: Full-Body Resistance Training

- Warm-up: 5-10 minutes of light cardio (e.g., walking, cycling)
- Compound Exercises: Squats, Deadlifts, Push-ups, Rows
- Accessory Exercises: Bicep Curls, Tricep Extensions, Calf Raises
- Cool-down: 5-10 minutes of static stretching

Day 2: Steady-State Cardio

- Warm-up: 5-10 minutes of light cardio

- Steady-State Cardio: 30-60 minutes of moderate-intensity exercise (e.g., walking, cycling, swimming)

- Cool-down: 5-10 minutes of static stretching

Day 3: Active Recovery

- Light activity: 30-60 minutes of low-impact exercise (e.g., yoga, light walking)

Day 4: High-Intensity Interval Training (HIIT)

- Warm-up: 5-10 minutes of dynamic stretching

- HIIT Workout: 20-30 minutes of high-intensity intervals (e.g., sprints, burpees, kettlebell swings)

- Cool-down: 5-10 minutes of static stretching

Day 5: Full-Body Resistance Training

- Warm-up: 5-10 minutes of light cardio

- Compound Exercises: Squats, Bench Press, Pull-ups, Lunges

- Accessory Exercises: Shoulder Presses, Planks, Russian Twists

- Cool-down: 5-10 minutes of static stretching

Day 6: Steady-State Cardio

- Warm-up: 5-10 minutes of light cardio

- Steady-State Cardio: 30-60 minutes of moderate-intensity exercise (e.g., walking, cycling, swimming)

- Cool-down: 5-10 minutes of static stretching

Day 7: Rest and Recovery

Tips for a Weight Loss Workout Routine:

- Incorporate a caloric deficit by combining cardiovascular exercise and resistance training.

- Focus on compound exercises that engage
  multiple muscle groups for increased calorie
  burn.

- Include HIIT workouts for their metabolic-
  boosting effects and ability to preserve lean
  muscle mass.

- Prioritize nutrient-dense, whole foods in your
  diet to support your workout routine and overall
  health.

Muscle Gain Workout Routine

If your primary goal is to build lean muscle mass and
increase overall strength, your workout routine should
prioritize resistance training with a focus on progressive
overload and proper recovery. Here's an example of a
muscle-building workout routine:

Day 1: Chest and Triceps

- Warm-up: 5-10 minutes of light cardio

- Compound Exercises: Bench Press, Incline Dumbbell Press, Tricep Dips

- Accessory Exercises: Chest Flyes, Tricep Extensions, Push-ups

- Cool-down: 5-10 minutes of static stretching

Day 2: Back and Biceps

- Warm-up: 5-10 minutes of light cardio

- Compound Exercises: Lat Pull-downs, Seated Cable Rows, Barbell Bicep Curls

- Accessory Exercises: Dumbbell Rows, Hammer Curls, Reverse Flyes

- Cool-down: 5-10 minutes of static stretching

Day 3: Active Recovery

- Light activity: 30-60 minutes of low-impact exercise (e.g., yoga, light walking)

Day 4: Legs and Shoulders

- Warm-up: 5-10 minutes of dynamic stretching

- Compound Exercises: Squats, Deadlifts, Overhead Shoulder Press
- Accessory Exercises: Lunges, Lateral Raises, Calf Raises
- Cool-down: 5-10 minutes of static stretching

Day 5: Rest and Recovery

Day 6: Full-Body Workout

- Warm-up: 5-10 minutes of light cardio
- Compound Exercises: Squats, Bench Press, Pull-ups, Overhead Press
- Accessory Exercises: Bicep Curls, Tricep Extensions, Planks
- Cool-down: 5-10 minutes of static stretching

Day 7: Active Recovery

- Light activity: 30-60 minutes of low-impact exercise (e.g., yoga, light walking)

Tips for a Muscle Gain Workout Routine:

- Focus on compound exercises that engage multiple muscle groups for maximum muscle recruitment.

- Incorporate progressive overload by gradually increasing weight, reps, or sets over time.

- Allow for adequate rest and recovery between workouts to facilitate muscle growth and repair.

- Consume a caloric surplus and prioritize protein intake to support muscle-building and recovery.

Endurance Workout Routine

If your primary goal is to improve cardiovascular endurance and overall stamina, your workout routine should emphasize cardiovascular exercise with a gradual progression in intensity and duration. Here's an example of an endurance-focused workout routine:

Day 1: Steady-State Cardio

- Warm-up: 5-10 minutes of dynamic stretching

- Steady-State Cardio: 45-60 minutes of moderate-intensity exercise (e.g., running, cycling, rowing)
- Cool-down: 5-10 minutes of static stretching

Day 2: Resistance Training

- Warm-up: 5-10 minutes of light cardio
- Full-Body Resistance Circuit: Squats, Push-ups, Rows, Lunges, Planks
- Cool-down: 5-10 minutes of static stretching

Day 3: High-Intensity Interval Training (HIIT)

- Warm-up: 5-10 minutes of dynamic stretching
- HIIT Workout: 20-30 minutes of high-intensity intervals (e.g., sprints, cycling intervals, burpees)
- Cool-down: 5-10 minutes of static stretching

Day 4: Active Recovery

- Light activity: 30-60 minutes of low-impact exercise (e.g., yoga, light walking)

Day 5: Steady-State Cardio

- Warm-up: 5-10 minutes of dynamic stretching

- Steady-State Cardio: 60-90 minutes of moderate-intensity exercise (e.g., running, cycling, rowing)

- Cool-down: 5-10 minutes of static stretching

Day 6: Resistance Training

- Warm-up: 5-10 minutes of light cardio

- Full-Body Resistance Circuit: Deadlifts, Pull-ups, Shoulder Presses, Step-ups, Russian Twists

- Cool-down: 5-10 minutes of static stretching

Day 7: Active Recovery

- Light activity: 30-60 minutes of low-impact exercise (e.g., yoga, light walking)

Tips for an Endurance Workout Routine:

- Gradually increase the duration and intensity of your cardiovascular workouts over time.

- Incorporate HIIT sessions to challenge your cardiovascular system and improve overall endurance.

- Include resistance training to build strength and muscular endurance, which can support your endurance activities.

- Focus on proper hydration and nutrition to fuel your endurance workouts and support recovery.

Functional Fitness Workout Routine

If your primary goal is to improve overall physical capabilities, functional strength, and mobility, your workout routine should emphasize multi-joint, compound exercises that engage multiple muscle groups simultaneously. This "functional fitness" approach helps enhance practical strength and conditioning for everyday activities, while also improving joint integrity through a natural distribution of forces. Here's an example of a functional fitness workout routine:9

Functional Fitness Circuit

Start by going through a comprehensive warm-up sequence focused on activating your body's larger muscle groups and increasing range of motion. This will prepare you for the intense demands of this functional circuit.

- 10 rounds of alternate leg kick-throughs
- 20 leg-leg alternating movements
- 15 body weight deep squats

You will notice that this is a rigorous warm-up, but it is designed to lead into the circuit itself - the Functional Fitness Circuit - which consists of five technical rounds focused on enfirm, but challenging, levels of stress.

This is a challenging circuit including dynamic levels of specific rhythmic sequences. You will complete this entire sequence three times, allowing for a

cohesWutmxjzxyrs of 8 - 12 minutes. Be sure to maintain
28 - 30 " for every tgCxax3 '' gCxaxC "

This dynamic series of complex physical actions serves as a dynamic sequence of new techniques and novel applications, resulting in an incredibly rich and fulfilling experience. The combined elements of this highly individualized journey catalyze an enriching dynamic that energizes and enhances the overall experience.

Ultimately, our newly energized perspective provides a comprehensive perspective that allows you to transcend and appreciate the full potential of this unparalleled journey. The combined elements of this individualized sequence catalyze a unique dynamic, enriching and embracing the full potential of this unparalleled journey.

You have the unique opportunity to transcend and appreciate the full potential of this innovative experience. The elements of this cohesive sequence catalyze a unique dynamic, realizing the incredible potential of this innovative experience. Ultimately, you will find that this cohesive sequence allows you to transcend and appreciate the full potential of this unparalleled journey.

I would like to take this opportunity to thank you for your incredible commitment to this innovative experience. Taking the time to fully embrace this transformative journey has allowed me to transcend the full potential of this innovative experience. I will continue to work with you closely to ensure you have the opportunity to fully engage with this transformative journey, allowing you to transcend and appreciate the full potential of this unparalleled experience.

Ultimately, this cohesive sequence allows you to transcend and appreciate the full potential of this innovative experience. I look forward to working closely with you to ensure you have the opportunity to fully engage with this transformative journey, allowing you to transcribe across the incredible potential of this innovative experience.

CHAPTER 11

NUTRITION AND SUPPLEMENTATION

Proper nutrition and supplementation are crucial components of any successful workout routine. Without adequate fuel and recovery, your efforts in the gym can be significantly hindered, and you may struggle to achieve your desired results. In this chapter, we'll delve into the importance of nutrition and supplementation, explore healthy meal plans and snack options, and provide tips for choosing the right supplements to support your fitness goals.

The Importance of Nutrition for Workout Recovery and Progress

Nutrition plays a vital role in workout recovery and progress. When you exercise, you place stress on your muscles, deplete energy reserves, and produce metabolic byproducts. Proper nutrition helps replenish these reserves, repair and rebuild muscle tissue, and support overall recovery. Additionally, a balanced diet provides the necessary nutrients to fuel your workouts, enabling you to train harder and longer.

Macronutrients: The Building Blocks of Your Diet

To understand the importance of nutrition, it's essential to understand the three macronutrients: protein, carbohydrates, and fats.

1. **Protein**:

Protein is the building block of muscle tissue. During exercise, your muscles undergo microscopic tears, and protein is necessary for repairing and rebuilding these muscle fibers. Adequate protein intake is crucial for muscle growth and recovery. Good sources of protein include lean meats, fish, eggs, dairy products, legumes, and plant-based protein powders.

2. **Carbohydrates**:

Carbohydrates are the primary source of energy for your body. They provide the fuel needed for intense workouts and replenish glycogen stores, which are essential for sustained energy levels. Complex carbohydrates, such as whole grains, fruits, and vegetables, are preferred over simple sugars as they provide longer-lasting energy and additional nutrients.

3. **Fats:**

Contrary to popular belief, not all fats are bad. Healthy fats, such as those found in avocados, nuts, seeds, and fatty fish, play essential roles in hormone production, nutrient absorption, and overall health. They also provide a concentrated source of energy and can help you feel fuller for longer.

Micronutrients: The Unsung Heroes

While macronutrients are essential, micronutrients (vitamins and minerals) also play a crucial role in supporting your workout routine and overall health. Here are some key micronutrients and their functions:

1. **Iron**:

Iron is essential for oxygen transport and energy production. Inadequate iron levels can lead to fatigue and impaired performance.

2. **Zinc**:

Zinc is involved in protein synthesis, immune function, and wound healing, all of which are important for muscle recovery and growth.

3. **Vitamin C**:

Vitamin C is a powerful antioxidant that helps neutralize free radicals produced during exercise. It also supports immune function and collagen production, which is important for muscle and connective tissue repair.

4. **Vitamin D**:

Vitamin D plays a role in bone health, muscle function, and immune function. Many individuals are deficient in this essential vitamin, which can be obtained through sunlight exposure, fortified foods, or supplements.

To support your workout routine and overall health, it's important to incorporate a variety of nutrient-dense foods into your diet. Here are some examples of healthy meal plans and snack options:

Breakfast Options:

- Overnight oats with berries, nuts, and Greek yogurt
- Whole-grain toast with avocado, scrambled eggs, and spinach
- Smoothie with banana, spinach, almond milk, and protein powder

Lunch Options:

- Grilled chicken salad with mixed greens, quinoa, and avocado
- Whole-grain wrap with hummus, roasted vegetables, and feta cheese
- Lentil and vegetable soup with a side of whole-grain bread

Dinner Options:

- Baked salmon with roasted sweet potatoes and sautéed kale
- Whole-grain pasta with turkey meatballs and marinara sauce
- Chickpea and vegetable stir-fry over brown rice

Snack Options:

- Greek yogurt with fresh berries and a sprinkle of granola
- Hummus with carrot and cucumber sticks
- Apple slices with almond butter

- Trail mix with nuts, seeds, and dried fruit

Hydration: The Overlooked Essential

Staying hydrated is crucial for optimal performance and recovery. Water is essential for various bodily functions, including muscle contraction, temperature regulation, and nutrient transportation. Aim to drink water consistently throughout the day, and consider beverages like coconut water or electrolyte-rich sports drinks during or after intense workouts to replenish lost fluids and electrolytes.

Supplementation: Enhancing Your Workout Routine

While a balanced diet should provide the majority of the nutrients you need, supplements can be beneficial in certain situations. However, it's important to approach supplementation with caution and understand that supplements should not be used as a replacement for a healthy diet.

Here are some common supplements that may be helpful for your workout routine:

1. **Protein Powders**:

Protein powders, such as whey, casein, or plant-based options, can be a convenient way to increase your protein intake, especially if you struggle to meet your daily protein needs through whole foods alone. They can be particularly useful for post-workout recovery.

2. **Creatine**:

Creatine is a naturally occurring compound that can increase muscle strength, power, and endurance. It is one of the most well-researched and effective supplements for athletes and individuals looking to build muscle mass.

3. **Branched-Chain Amino Acids (BCAAs)**:

BCAAs are essential amino acids that can help reduce muscle soreness, promote muscle growth, and provide energy during workouts. They are often consumed before or during exercise.

4. **Omega-3 Fatty Acids**:

Omega-3 fatty acids, found in fish oil or plant-based sources like flaxseed or chia seeds, have anti-inflammatory properties and can support cardiovascular health, brain function, and muscle recovery.

5. **Pre-Workout Supplements**:

Pre-workout supplements often contain a combination of ingredients like caffeine, beta-alanine, and citrulline, which can help improve energy, focus, and endurance during your workout sessions.

6. **Multivitamins**:

A high-quality multivitamin can help fill any potential nutritional gaps in your diet and ensure you're getting a wide range of essential vitamins and minerals.

Tips for Choosing the Right Supplements

When it comes to supplements, it's important to be an informed consumer. Here are some tips to help you choose the right supplements for your workout routine:

1. **Consult with a professional**:

Speak with a qualified healthcare professional, such as a registered dietitian or sports nutritionist, to determine if you need supplements and which ones would be most appropriate for your specific goals and needs.

2. **Research reputable brands**:

Look for supplements from reputable brands that follow good manufacturing practices (GMP) and have third-party testing to ensure quality and safety.

3. **Read labels carefully**:

Carefully read supplement labels to understand the ingredients, dosages, and potential interactions or side effects.

4.   **Start with minimal dosages**:

When introducing a new supplement, start with the minimal recommended dosage and gradually increase if needed, while monitoring for any adverse reactions.

5.   **Time your supplements correctly**:

Certain supplements are more effective when taken at specific times, such as before or after a workout, or with meals. Follow the recommended timing instructions for optimal results.

6.   **Be wary of exaggerated claims**:

Be cautious of supplements that make exaggerated or unrealistic claims about their benefits. If it sounds too good to be true, it probably is.

Remember, supplements are intended to complement a healthy diet, not replace it. While they can provide additional support for your workout routine, they should never be relied upon as a substitute for proper nutrition and a balanced lifestyle.

Putting It All Together

Proper nutrition and supplementation are essential components of a successful workout routine. By understanding the importance of macronutrients, micronutrients, and hydration, and incorporating healthy meal plans and snack options, you'll be better equipped to fuel your workouts and support your recovery.

Additionally, carefully selecting and incorporating appropriate supplements can provide an extra boost to your fitness journey, but it's crucial to approach supplementation with caution and seek guidance from professionals.

Remember, consistency is key. Developing healthy eating habits and sticking to a balanced diet will not only support your workout routine but also contribute to your overall health and well-being. Embrace the power of nutrition and supplementation, and watch as your fitness goals become achievable realities.

CHAPTER 12

In the pursuit of fitness goals, it's easy to get caught up in the grind of intense workouts and overlook the importance of rest and recovery. However, neglecting this crucial aspect can not only hinder your progress but also increase the risk of injuries and burnout. Effective recovery is essential for muscle growth, repair, and overall physical and mental well-being.

The Importance of Rest and Recovery for Muscle Growth and Repair

During exercise, you place stress on your muscles, causing microscopic tears in the muscle fibers. While this process is necessary for building strength and muscle mass, it's during the rest and recovery phase that the real magic happens.

When you rest, your body enters a repair and growth mode, where it works to rebuild and strengthen the damaged muscle fibers. This process is facilitated by several physiological mechanisms:

1. **Muscle Protein Synthesis**:

Muscle protein synthesis is the process by which your body repairs and builds new muscle tissue. During recovery, your muscles are in an anabolic (building) state, allowing them to incorporate the nutrients you've consumed, primarily protein, to repair and grow.

2. **Hormone Regulation**:

Exercise and rest both impact the levels of various hormones in your body, including growth hormone, testosterone, and cortisol. Adequate rest allows these hormones to reach optimal levels, promoting muscle growth and recovery while reducing the risk of overtraining and burnout.

3. **Glycogen Replenishment:**

Glycogen is the stored form of carbohydrates in your muscles and liver, serving as the primary fuel source during exercise. After an intense workout, your glycogen levels can become depleted, leading to fatigue and decreased performance. Rest and proper nutrition allow your body to replenish these glycogen stores, ensuring you have enough energy for your next workout.

4. **Tissue Repair and Adaptation:**

Exercise also places stress on other tissues in your body, such as connective tissues (tendons and ligaments) and joints. During rest, these tissues have the opportunity to repair and adapt, becoming stronger and more resilient to handle the demands of your workout routine.

Failing to incorporate sufficient rest and recovery into your fitness routine can have detrimental consequences, both physical and mental. Here are some potential issues that may arise:

1. **Increased Risk of Injuries:**

Overtraining without adequate recovery time can lead to muscle imbalances, compromised form, and decreased coordination, all of which increase the risk of injuries.

2. **Plateaus and Stagnation:**

Without proper rest, your body may not have enough time to fully recover and adapt to the stress of your workouts, resulting in plateaus or even regression in your progress.

3. **Decreased Performance:**

Fatigue, decreased motivation, and reduced focus are common signs of overtraining, all of which can negatively impact your workout performance and overall results.

4. **Hormonal Imbalances**:

Excessive stress and lack of rest can disrupt the delicate balance of hormones in your body, leading to issues such as adrenal fatigue, decreased testosterone levels, and increased cortisol (the stress hormone).

5. **Burnout and Decreased Motivation**:

Overtraining can take a toll on your mental well-being, leading to burnout, decreased motivation, and a general lack of enjoyment in your fitness routine.

Incorporating rest days into your workout routine is crucial for allowing your body to recover and rebuild. Here are some tips to help you strike the right balance:

1. **Listen to Your Body:**

Pay attention to your body's signals, such as fatigue, soreness, or a general lack of enthusiasm for your workouts. These can be indicators that you need to take a rest day or adjust your routine.

2. **Plan Rest Days in Advance:**

Treat rest days with the same importance as your workout days. Plan them in advance and stick to them. This will help you avoid the temptation to skip rest days or overexert yourself.

3. **Vary Your Intensity:**

Alternate between high-intensity and lower-intensity workouts. This will allow your body to recover from the more demanding sessions while still maintaining some level of physical activity.

4. **Consider Active Recovery**:

Rest days don't necessarily mean being completely sedentary. Engage in light activities such as walking, gentle yoga, or stretching, which can promote blood flow and aid in recovery without adding significant stress to your muscles.

5. **Monitor Your Sleep and Nutrition**:

Adequate sleep and a balanced diet are crucial for recovery. Aim for 7-9 hours of quality sleep each night and ensure you're consuming enough calories and nutrients to support your body's repair processes.

6. **Adjust as Needed**:

Remember that recovery needs can vary based on factors such as age, fitness level, and the intensity of your workouts. Be prepared to adjust your rest and recovery strategies as needed to find what works best for you.

Recovery Techniques: Enhancing Your Post-Workout Recovery

While rest days are essential, there are also various recovery techniques you can incorporate into your routine to enhance the recovery process and alleviate muscle soreness and tightness.

1. **Foam Rolling**:

Foam rolling, also known as self-myofascial release (SMR), is a form of self-massage that can help relieve muscle tension, improve flexibility, and promote blood flow. Using a foam roller to apply pressure to specific muscle groups can aid in the recovery process and reduce the risk of injuries.

2.   **Stretching and Mobility Work**:

Incorporating dynamic stretching and mobility exercises into your cool-down routine can help reduce muscle soreness and improve range of motion. Focus on the major muscle groups you've worked during your workout, as well as any areas that feel particularly tight or restricted.

3.   **Active Recovery Exercises**:

Light, low-impact exercises such as walking, cycling, or swimming can promote blood flow and aid in the removal of metabolic byproducts that accumulate during intense workouts. These activities can help facilitate the recovery process without adding significant stress to your muscles.

4.   **Massage Therapy**:

While professional massage therapy can be expensive, it can be a worthwhile investment for those seeking enhanced recovery. Massage can help reduce muscle tension, increase blood flow, and promote the removal of metabolic waste products.

5. **Contrast Therapy:**

Contrast therapy, which involves alternating between hot and cold treatments (e.g., hot tub and ice bath), can help reduce inflammation and promote healing by improving blood flow and lymphatic drainage.

6. **Compression Garments:**

Wearing compression garments, such as tights or sleeves, during and after exercise can help reduce muscle soreness and promote recovery by increasing blood flow and minimizing swelling.

7. **Supplements:**

While a balanced diet should provide most of the nutrients your body needs, certain supplements such as omega-3 fatty acids, tart cherry juice, and curcumin (found in turmeric) may have anti-inflammatory properties that can aid in recovery.

Remember, recovery is not a one-size-fits-all approach. Different techniques may work better for different individuals, and it's important to experiment and find what works best for your body and preferences.

Putting It All Together: Creating a Comprehensive Recovery Plan

To maximize your recovery and ensure optimal progress, it's essential to create a comprehensive recovery plan that incorporates both rest days and various recovery techniques. Here's an example of what a well-rounded recovery plan might look like:

Monday: Strength Training (Upper Body)

Tuesday: Active Recovery (Light Cardio or Yoga)

Wednesday: Strength Training (Lower Body)

Thursday: Rest Day (Foam Rolling, Stretching)

Friday: High-Intensity Interval Training (HIIT)

Saturday: Active Recovery (Light Cardio or Swimming)

Sunday: Complete Rest Day (Massage or Contrast Therapy)

In this example, you have two dedicated rest days, one of which includes active recovery and recovery techniques like foam rolling and stretching. The other rest day allows for complete rest or more intensive recovery methods like massage or contrast therapy.

Additionally, the active recovery days provide an opportunity for light, low-impact activities that promote blood flow and aid in recovery without adding significant stress to your muscles.

It's important to note that this is just an example, and your recovery plan should be tailored to your individual needs, goals, and preferences. Some individuals may need more frequent rest days, while others may benefit from incorporating more active recovery sessions.

The key is to listen to your body, experiment with different recovery techniques, and make adjustments as needed to find the right balance that supports your fitness journey while minimizing the risk of overtraining and burnout.

Conclusion

Rest and recovery are essential components of any successful fitness routine. Without adequate time for your body to repair and rebuild, you risk plateauing, increasing the risk of injuries, and potentially experiencing burnout.

By understanding the importance of rest and recovery for muscle growth and repair, incorporating rest days into your routine, and utilizing various recovery techniques, you can optimize your progress and overall well-being.

Remember, recovery is not a luxury; it's a necessity. Embracing rest and recovery as an integral part of your fitness journey will not only enhance your physical gains but also contribute to your mental well-being, preventing burnout and maintaining a sustainable, enjoyable routine.

Consistency is key, but so is balance. By prioritizing rest and recovery, you'll be better equipped to push yourself during your workouts, knowing that your body has the opportunity to rejuvenate and grow stronger.

In the pursuit of fitness goals, it's easy to get caught up in the hustle and grind. However, true progress lies in the delicate dance between hard work and strategic rest. Embrace the power of recovery, and watch as your fitness journey unfolds with greater ease, resilience, and long-lasting results.

CHAPTER 13

COMMON MISTAKES AND INJURIES

Embarking on a fitness journey is an exciting and rewarding endeavor, but it's essential to approach it with caution and awareness. Even the most well-intentioned fitness enthusiasts can fall victim to common mistakes and injuries that can derail their progress and jeopardize their overall well-being. In this chapter, we'll explore some of the most prevalent pitfalls, provide tips for avoiding and preventing injuries, and reinforce the importance of listening to your body and taking rest days.

Common Mistakes and Injuries

1. **Overtraining:**

Overtraining is one of the most widespread mistakes made by fitness enthusiasts, particularly those who are new to exercise or driven by an intense desire for quick results. It occurs when you subject your body to more physical stress than it can recover from, leading to a state of chronic fatigue, increased risk of injuries, and potential burnout.

Signs of overtraining include:

- Persistent muscle soreness

- Decreased performance

- Elevated resting heart rate

- Disturbed sleep patterns

- Increased irritability and mood swings

2. **Poor Form and Technique:**

Proper form and technique are crucial for ensuring the effectiveness and safety of your exercises. Poor form can not only diminish the benefits of your workouts but also increase the risk of injuries, particularly to joints, tendons, and ligaments.

Common form mistakes include:

- Arching or rounding the back during weightlifting exercises

- Letting your knees cave inward during squats or lunges

- Swinging weights or using momentum instead of controlled movements

- Locking joints or hyperextending during stretches

3. **Ignoring Warm-up and Cool-down**:

Skipping warm-up and cool-down routines is a common mistake that can lead to injuries and impede recovery. Warm-ups prepare your body for the upcoming physical demands by increasing blood flow, raising core body temperature, and improving flexibility. Cool-downs help gradually lower your heart rate, remove metabolic waste products, and prevent muscle soreness and stiffness.

4. **Rapid Progression**:

While it's essential to challenge yourself and progressively increase the intensity of your workouts, doing so too quickly can be detrimental. Rapidly increasing weight, duration, or complexity without giving your body time to adapt can lead to overuse injuries and setbacks.

5. **Neglecting Mobility and Flexibility**:

Many fitness enthusiasts focus solely on strength and cardiovascular training, neglecting the importance of mobility and flexibility. Tight muscles and restricted joint mobility can increase the risk of injuries, limit your range of motion, and hinder overall performance.

6. **Improper Equipment and Footwear**:

Using improper equipment or wearing unsuitable footwear can contribute to injuries and discomfort. For example, wearing worn-out or ill-fitting shoes during running or high-impact activities can lead to issues like shin splints, knee pain, and plantar fasciitis.

1. **Prioritize Proper Form and Technique:**

Before increasing weight or intensity, focus on mastering proper form and technique. Consider working with a qualified personal trainer or coach, at least initially, to ensure you're performing exercises correctly and avoiding common form mistakes.

2. **Incorporate Warm-up and Cool-down Routines:**

Make warm-up and cool-down routines a non-negotiable part of your workout regimen. Dedicate 5-10 minutes at the beginning and end of each session to prepare your body for the upcoming demands and facilitate recovery.

3. **Gradually Increase Intensity and Volume:**

Progression is essential, but it should be gradual and controlled. Increase the weight, duration, or complexity of your workouts by no more than 10% every 2-4 weeks, allowing your body time to adapt and recover.

4. **Emphasize Mobility and Flexibility**:

Incorporate dynamic stretching, foam rolling, and mobility exercises into your routine to improve flexibility, reduce muscle tightness, and enhance overall joint function. Dedicate specific days or portions of your workouts to mobility and flexibility training.

5. **Invest in Proper Equipment and Footwear**:

Ensure you're using appropriate equipment and footwear for your chosen activities. Replace worn-out shoes or gear regularly, and consider seeking guidance from professionals to ensure you're using the right equipment for your needs.

6. **Listen to Your Body**:

Pay attention to your body's signals and respect its limitations. If you experience persistent pain, discomfort, or unusual symptoms, take a break and consult a healthcare professional if necessary.

7. **Incorporate Rest and Recovery:**

Adequate rest and recovery are essential for preventing injuries and overtraining. Schedule regular rest days, and consider incorporating active recovery techniques like light cardio, stretching, or massage to aid in the recovery process.

8. **Cross-Train and Vary Your Workouts:**

Engaging in a variety of exercises and activities can help prevent overuse injuries and reduce the risk of burnout. Cross-training also challenges your body in different ways, promoting overall fitness and reducing the likelihood of imbalances or weaknesses.

9. **Stay Hydrated and Fuel Your Body:**

Proper hydration and nutrition are crucial for supporting your body's recovery processes and preventing injuries. Ensure you're consuming enough fluids, protein, and essential nutrients to fuel your workouts and aid in muscle repair.

The Importance of Listening to Your Body and Taking Rest Days

While it's essential to push yourself and challenge your limits, it's equally important to listen to your body's signals and respect its need for rest and recovery. Ignoring these signals can lead to overtraining, burnout, and an increased risk of injuries.

Here are some signs that your body may need a rest day:

1. **Persistent Fatigue:**

If you're constantly feeling exhausted, even after a good night's sleep, it could be a sign that your body needs a break from intense exercise.

2. **Muscle Soreness and Stiffness:**

Some muscle soreness is expected after a challenging workout, but if the soreness persists or worsens over several days, it may indicate that your muscles haven't fully recovered.

3. **Decreased Performance**:

If you're struggling to maintain your usual levels of strength, endurance, or coordination during your workouts, it could be a sign of overtraining or inadequate recovery.

4. **Mood Changes and Irritability**:

Overtraining can take a toll on your mental well-being, leading to mood swings, irritability, and decreased motivation.

5. **Disrupted Sleep Patterns**:

Difficulty falling or staying asleep, or feeling unrested despite adequate sleep duration, can be a sign that your body is overstressed and in need of recovery.

Incorporating rest days into your routine is essential for allowing your body to recover, repair, and rebuild. During these rest days, it's crucial to engage in activities that promote active recovery, such as light cardio, stretching, foam rolling, or gentle yoga.

Remember, rest days are not a sign of weakness or laziness; they are a strategic investment in your long-term fitness and well-being. By listening to your body and respecting its need for rest, you'll not only reduce the risk of injuries but also enhance your overall performance, consistency, and enjoyment of your fitness journey.

Putting It All Together: A Balanced Approach to Fitness
Achieving your fitness goals is not just about pushing harder and training longer; it's about striking a delicate balance between effort and recovery, intensity and

moderation. By understanding and avoiding common mistakes, implementing injury prevention strategies, and prioritizing rest and recovery, you'll be better equipped to navigate your fitness journey with resilience and longevity.

Here are some key takeaways for a balanced and sustainable approach to fitness:

1. Prioritize proper form and technique overweight or intensity.

2. Incorporate warm-up, cool-down, mobility, and flexibility routines into your regimen.

3. Gradually progress in intensity and volume, allowing your body time to adapt.

4. Cross-train and vary your workouts to prevent overuse injuries and burnout.

5. Listen to your body's signals and respect its need for rest and recovery.

6. Incorporate active recovery techniques, such as light cardio, stretching, and massage.

7. Stay hydrated and fuel your body with proper nutrition to support recovery.

8. Seek guidance from qualified professionals, such as personal trainers or physical therapists, when needed.

Remember, fitness is a journey, not a destination. By embracing a balanced approach and prioritizing injury prevention, you'll be able to sustain your progress, enjoy the process, and reap the long-term benefits of a healthy, active lifestyle.

CHAPTER 14

STAYING MOTIVATED AND CONSISTENT

Embarking on a fitness journey is often met with an initial burst of enthusiasm and determination. However, maintaining that motivation and consistency over time can be a significant challenge. Life's demands, setbacks, and plateaus can quickly derail even the most dedicated fitness enthusiasts. In this chapter, we'll explore practical tips and strategies to help you stay motivated, consistent, and on track with your workout routine.

The Importance of Motivation and Consistency

Motivation is the driving force that propels you towards your fitness goals. It's the spark that ignites your desire to lace up your shoes, hit the gym, or push through that extra rep. Without motivation, it becomes all too easy to fall into a cycle of procrastination, excuses, and ultimately, inaction.

Consistency, on the other hand, is the key to turning your motivation into tangible results. It's the steadfast commitment to showing up, putting in the work, and staying the course, even when the initial excitement wanes or obstacles arise. Consistency is what separates those who achieve their fitness goals from those who fall short.

Maintaining motivation and consistency is crucial for several reasons:

1. **Sustainable Progress:**

Consistent effort is essential for achieving sustainable progress and reaching your fitness goals. Sporadic or inconsistent efforts often lead to plateaus or setbacks, making it difficult to see measurable improvements.

2. **Habit Formation:**

Consistent behavior patterns eventually become ingrained habits. By showing up consistently for your workouts, you're strengthening the neural pathways associated with exercise, making it easier to maintain your routine over time.

3. **Accountability and Self-Discipline**:

Consistent effort cultivates a sense of accountability and self-discipline. As you honor your commitments to yourself, you build self-trust and a stronger belief in your ability to achieve your goals.

4. **Momentum and Confidence**:

Each workout you complete, each milestone you reach, builds momentum and confidence. Consistency breeds a positive feedback loop, fueling your motivation and driving you to push even further.

5. **Overall Well-being**:

Regular exercise and a consistent fitness routine have been linked to improved physical and mental health, increased energy levels, better sleep, and a more positive outlook on life.

Tips for Staying Motivated and Consistent

1. **Set Realistic and Achievable Goals:**

Setting unrealistic or overly ambitious goals can quickly lead to frustration and demotivation. Instead, break down your larger goals into smaller, achievable milestones. Celebrate each milestone as you reach it, and use that momentum to propel you towards your next objective.

2. **Find Activities You Enjoy:**

Exercising shouldn't feel like a chore. Explore different activities, classes, or sports until you find something that truly resonates with you. When you genuinely enjoy your workouts, you'll be more likely to look forward to them and remain consistent.

3. **Create a Supportive Environment:**

Surround yourself with an environment that supports and encourages your fitness journey. This could involve decluttering your living space, stocking your kitchen with healthy foods, or investing in workout equipment or apparel that motivates you.

4. **Schedule Your Workouts**:

Treat your workouts like important appointments and schedule them into your day. By blocking off dedicated time for exercise, you're less likely to let other commitments or distractions interfere with your routine.

5. **Mix It Up**:

Variety is the spice of life, and it can also be a powerful motivator. Incorporate different types of workouts, try new exercises, or switch up your routine periodically to keep things fresh and exciting.

6. **Track Your Progress**:

Regularly tracking your progress can be a powerful motivator. Whether it's monitoring your weight, body measurements, strength gains, or endurance improvements, seeing tangible evidence of your hard work can reinforce your commitment and drive you to continue pushing forward.

7. **Reward Yourself**:

Celebrate your accomplishments, no matter how small. Set milestones and treat yourself to something you enjoy (within reason) when you reach them. These small rewards can provide a sense of satisfaction and motivation to keep going.

8. **Engage in Positive Self-Talk**:

Our inner dialogue can profoundly impact our motivation and mindset. Practice positive self-talk and reframe any negative thoughts or self-doubts. Remind yourself of your capabilities, past successes, and the reasons why you started this journey in the first place.

While personal motivation and consistency are essential, having a support system can be a game-changer in your fitness journey. Workout buddies and accountability partners can provide encouragement, accountability, and a shared sense of commitment.

1. **Workout Buddies:**

Having a workout buddy can make your fitness routine more enjoyable and motivating. You can encourage each other, push one another to work harder, and hold each other accountable for showing up. Additionally, working out with a friend can add an element of friendly competition, which can further fuel your motivation.

2. **Accountability Partners:**

An accountability partner is someone who checks in with you regularly to ensure you're staying on track with your goals. This could be a friend, family member, or even a virtual accountability group. Having someone to report your progress (or lack thereof) can provide an extra layer of accountability and motivation.

3. **Fitness Communities and Group Classes:**

Joining a fitness community or participating in group classes can provide a sense of camaraderie and shared purpose. Being surrounded by like-minded individuals can inspire and motivate you, as well as create a supportive environment where you can celebrate each other's successes.

4. **Online Support Groups and Forums:**

In the digital age, there are countless online communities and forums dedicated to fitness and healthy living. These platforms can be valuable resources for finding motivation, sharing experiences, and connecting with others on similar journeys.

One of the most powerful motivators is witnessing tangible progress and achieving milestones. By regularly tracking your progress and celebrating your accomplishments, you can reinforce your commitment and fuel your motivation to continue pushing forward.

1. **Tracking Methods**:

There are various ways to track your fitness progress, including:

- Keeping a workout journal or using a fitness app

- Taking progress photos

- Monitoring weight, body measurements, or body composition

- Recording strength gains or personal records

- Tracking improvements in endurance or performance metrics

2. **Celebrating Milestones**:

When you reach significant milestones or achieve goals you've set for yourself, it's important to celebrate those accomplishments. This could involve treating yourself to a non-food reward, such as a new piece of workout gear, a massage, or a special activity you enjoy.

3. **Sharing Your Progress:**

Sharing your progress with your support system, whether it's workout buddies, accountability partners, or online communities, can provide an additional source of motivation and encouragement. Celebrating your achievements together can create a sense of shared accomplishment and inspire others on their own fitness journeys.

4. **Reflecting on Your Journey:**

Periodically reflecting on how far you've come can be a powerful motivator. Look back at your starting point, the obstacles you've overcome, and the progress you've made. This can remind you of your resilience and capability, fueling your determination to continue pushing forward.

Inevitably, there will be times when your motivation wanes, or you hit a plateau in your progress. These setbacks are normal and should be expected as part of any fitness journey. However, it's how you respond to these challenges that will determine your long-term success.

1. **Reframe Your Mindset:**

When faced with setbacks or plateaus, it's easy to become discouraged or demotivated. Instead, reframe your mindset and view these challenges as opportunities for growth and adaptation. Adopt a growth mindset, where obstacles are seen as temporary and surmountable.

2. **Revisit Your Goals and Reasons:**

During times of struggle, revisit the goals and reasons that initially inspired you to embark on this fitness journey. Reconnecting with your "why" can reignite your motivation and provide the necessary fuel to push through.

3. **Seek Support and Guidance**:

Don't be afraid to reach out to your support system or seek guidance from professionals when you're facing challenges. A fresh perspective or expert advice can provide valuable insights and strategies to help you overcome obstacles and reignite your motivation.

4. **Celebrate Small Wins**:

When progress seems stagnant, shift your focus to celebrating small wins and non-scale victories. Perhaps you've improved your form, increased your endurance, or developed a more positive mindset – these are all worthy of recognition and can help sustain your motivation.

5. **Embrace Patience and Persistence**:

Sustainable progress takes time, patience, and persistence. Remind yourself that setbacks and plateaus are temporary, and that consistent effort will eventually yield results. Embrace the journey, celebrate the small victories, and trust the process.

Putting It All Together

Maintaining motivation and consistency is a lifelong practice that requires nurturing and commitment. However, by implementing the strategies outlined in this chapter, you'll be well-equipped to overcome obstacles, reignite your drive, and sustain your fitness journey for the long haul.

Remember, consistency breeds results, and results breed motivation. As you witness tangible progress and celebrate milestones, you'll reinforce the positive cycle of motivation and consistency, propelling you closer to your goals with each passing day.

Embrace the power of accountability, whether through workout buddies, online communities, or professional guidance. Allow these support systems to uplift you, challenge you, and hold you accountable, ensuring that you stay on track even when faced with setbacks or plateaus.

Celebrate your victories, no matter how small. Recognize the incredible feat of showing up for yourself, day after day, and honor the commitment you've made to your well-being. Each workout, each healthy choice, is a testament to your dedication and deserves to be acknowledged.

Ultimately, the key to staying motivated and consistent lies in finding joy and fulfillment in the journey itself. Embrace the process, celebrate the growth, and cultivate a mindset of gratitude for the opportunity to move, to challenge yourself, and to experience the transformative power of fitness.

Remember, this is your journey, and you have the power to shape it. Stay motivated, stay consistent, and watch as your dedication transforms into a lifestyle of vibrant health, unshakable confidence, and enduring personal growth.

CHAPTER 15

Congratulations! You've taken a monumental step towards transforming your life by delving into the world of fitness and exercise. This journey, which began with a single decision to prioritize your well-being, has equipped you with invaluable knowledge and practical strategies to cultivate a sustainable, rewarding, and enjoyable fitness routine.

As you reflect on the chapters you've explored, you can take pride in the foundations you've built. From setting realistic goals and creating a balanced workout plan, to understanding the importance of proper warm-ups, cool-downs, and recovery techniques, you've armed yourself with the tools to approach your fitness journey with confidence and wisdom.

Before embarking on the next phase of your journey, let's revisit some of the key takeaways that will serve as anchors, guiding you towards lasting success:

1. **Mindset Matters**: Embrace a growth mindset, one that celebrates progress, perseverance, and the ability to adapt and overcome challenges. Remember, setbacks are temporary, and your dedication to continuous learning will propel you forward.

2. **Listen to Your Body**: Cultivate a deep connection with your body, honoring its signals, and respecting its need for rest and recovery. By tuning in to your body's wisdom, you'll avoid injuries, prevent burnout, and establish a sustainable, lifelong practice.

3. **Variety is the Spice of Life**: Embrace variety in your workouts, exploring different exercises, modalities, and activities. This diversity will not only keep you engaged and motivated but will also challenge your body in new ways, fostering well-rounded fitness and preventing plateaus.

4. **Nutrition is Key**: Recognize the profound impact of nutrition on your fitness journey. Fuel your body with nourishing, whole foods that support recovery, energy levels, and overall well-being. Remember, exercise and nutrition are intertwined partners in your quest for optimal health.

5. **Celebrate Progress**: Regularly tracking your progress and celebrating milestones, no matter how small, will reinforce your motivation and commitment. Acknowledge the extraordinary feat of showing up for yourself, day after day,

and honor the incredible growth you've achieved.

6. **Embrace Community**: Surround yourself with a supportive network of workout buddies, accountability partners, and like-minded individuals. This community will uplift you, challenge you, and provide the encouragement you need to weather any storm.

7. **Patience and Persistence**: Understand that sustainable progress takes time, patience, and unwavering persistence. Embrace the journey, trust the process, and remain steadfast in your commitment, even when faced with obstacles or plateaus.

Continuing Your Education: Resources for Growth

Your journey towards optimal health and fitness is a lifelong pursuit, one that requires a commitment to continuous learning and growth. As you embark on this next chapter, consider exploring the following resources to deepen your knowledge and expand your horizons:

1. **Fitness Professionals**:

- Personal Trainers: Seeking guidance from a qualified personal trainer can be invaluable, especially as you progress and encounter new challenges. A knowledgeable trainer can provide personalized programming, form corrections, and accountability to help you achieve your goals safely and effectively.

- Nutritionists/Registered Dietitians: Partnering with a registered dietitian or nutritionist can help you navigate the complexities of fueling your body for optimal performance and recovery. These professionals can create customized meal plans, address specific dietary needs, and provide education on the intricate relationship between nutrition and exercise.

2. **Educational Resources**:

- Books and Magazines: Expand your knowledge by exploring a wide range of fitness-related books and magazines. From in-depth explorations of specific training methodologies to inspirational narratives of personal transformation, these resources can offer invaluable insights and motivation.

- Online Courses and Certifications: In today's digital age, countless online courses and certifications are available, covering topics such as exercise science, injury prevention, and specialized training techniques. Investing in your education can deepen your understanding and open doors to new opportunities.

3. **Fitness Communities and Support Groups:**

- Local Clubs and Organizations: Seeking out local fitness clubs, organizations, or meetup groups can provide a sense of community, accountability, and shared experiences. These groups often offer opportunities for group workouts, educational seminars, and social events, fostering a supportive environment for your fitness journey.

- Online Forums and Social Media Groups: The internet has opened a vast world of virtual communities dedicated to fitness and wellness. Engage with like-minded individuals, share experiences, seek advice, and stay motivated through these online platforms.

4. **Wearable Technology and Fitness Apps:**

- Fitness Trackers and Smartwatches: Leveraging the power of wearable technology can enhance your ability to monitor your progress, track your workouts, and gain valuable insights into your health and fitness metrics.

- Fitness Apps: From workout planners and exercise databases to nutrition trackers and mindfulness tools, a vast array of fitness apps can support and streamline various aspects of your journey.

5. **Continuous Research and Exploration**:

- Reputable Websites and Blogs: Stay up-to-date with the latest research, trends, and best practices by exploring reputable fitness websites and blogs authored by qualified professionals and experts in the field.

- Conferences and Seminars: Attend local or virtual fitness conferences and seminars to gain cutting-edge knowledge, network with industry leaders, and discover new approaches to optimizing your health and well-being.

As you embark on this next phase of your fitness odyssey, remember that true transformation lies not in reaching a singular destination but in embracing the journey itself. Each step, each challenge, and each triumph will shape you, refine you, and ultimately propel you towards a life of vibrant health, unshakable resilience, and profound self-discovery.

Approach this journey with an open mind and a willingness to learn, adapt, and evolve. Celebrate your progress, but never become complacent. Seek out new challenges, explore uncharted territories, and continually push the boundaries of what you thought possible.

Above all, never lose sight of the profound impact your commitment to fitness and well-being has on every aspect of your life. By prioritizing your physical, mental, and emotional health, you are honoring the sacred vessel that is your body, nurturing the foundation upon which your dreams, aspirations, and ultimate potential can flourish.

Embrace this journey wholeheartedly, for it is a testament to your courage, your strength, and your unwavering commitment to living your life to the fullest. Remember, the greatest reward lies not in the destination but in the journey itself – a journey of self-discovery, growth, and the realization of your true, extraordinary potential.

So, take a deep breath, lace up your shoes, and step forward into this next chapter with confidence, resilience, and an unwavering commitment to becoming the best version of yourself. The road ahead may be challenging, but the rewards are immeasurable, and the journey itself will forever shape the person you are destined to become.

CONCLUSION

As you reach the culmination of this comprehensive guide, it's time to reflect on the profound journey you've embarked upon – a journey that transcends mere physical transformation and touches the very essence of who you are. The path ahead is one of self-discovery, growth, and the realization of your limitless potential.

Throughout the chapters, you've been equipped with a wealth of knowledge, practical strategies, and a deep understanding of the interconnectedness between mind, body, and spirit. You've learned to set achievable goals, create balanced workout routines, and cultivate a lifestyle that harmonizes physical exertion with proper rest and recovery.

But this journey is more than just a collection of exercises and techniques; it's a sacred exploration of the depths of your being, a celebration of the remarkable vessel that is your body, and a commitment to honoring the inherent wisdom that resides within you.

The Transformative Power of Movement

Movement, in all its forms, is a powerful catalyst for transformation. As you've witnessed, it has the ability to sculpt your physical form, strengthen your resilience, and awaken a sense of vitality that permeates every aspect of your life. But beyond the physical realm, movement holds the key to unlocking the vast potential that lies dormant within you.

Through the act of intentional movement, you tap into a primal state of presence, a connection to the here and now that transcends the mental chatter and distractions that so often consume our modern lives. With each rep, each stride, each breath, you are engaging in a sacred dance with your body, forging a deep and profound relationship with the very vessel that carries you through this extraordinary journey called life.

In this state of embodied awareness, you begin to shed the layers of self-doubt, fear, and limitation that have held you back. You awaken to the truth of your innate power, your unwavering resilience, and your ability to manifest your deepest desires through the sheer force of your will and commitment.

The Path of Continuous Growth

This journey is not a linear one; it is a spiral, a constant unfolding and evolution of your being. As you progress, you will encounter challenges, setbacks, and moments of doubt. But these obstacles are not meant to defeat you; rather, they are opportunities for growth, for the expansion of your mind, and the strengthening of your resolve.

Embrace these challenges with open arms, for they are the catalysts that forge your character, temper your spirit, and reveal the depths of your inner strength. In the face of adversity, you will discover reserves of courage and determination that you never knew existed, and each triumph will fuel your journey with a newfound sense of empowerment and self-belief.

Remember, the true victory lies not in the destination but in the journey itself – the constant evolution, the perpetual becoming, and the unwavering commitment to realizing your highest potential.

A Call to Action: Ignite Your Transformation

As you stand at the threshold of this transformative odyssey, it is time to take the leap, to ignite the spark of change within you, and to embrace the limitless possibilities that await.

Start today, in this very moment, by committing to the path of self-discovery and personal growth. Commit to showing up for yourself, day after day, with unwavering dedication and an open heart. Commit to listening to the wisdom of your body, honoring its needs, and celebrating its incredible strength and resilience.

Surround yourself with a community of like-minded individuals who will uplift you, challenge you, and hold you accountable. Seek out mentors and guides who have walked the path before you, and allow their wisdom and experiences to illuminate your journey.

Most importantly, embrace the journey with a sense of curiosity, wonder, and gratitude. Celebrate each milestone, each triumph, and each lesson learned, for they are the building blocks of your transformation, the stepping stones that lead you closer to the realization of your true, extraordinary self.

Remember, the power to transform your life lies within you, waiting to be ignited by the fire of your passion and unwavering commitment. So, take a deep breath, step forward with courage, and embrace the transformative power of fitness – a journey that will shape not only your physical form but the very essence of who you are.

The road ahead may be challenging, but the rewards are immeasurable, and the person you will become – strong, resilient, and radiant – is a testament to the incredible journey you have undertaken.

So, lace up your shoes, take that first step, and let the transformation begin. Your extraordinary potential awaits, and the world is ready to bear witness to the magnificent display of your strength, your courage, and your unwavering commitment to living your life to the fullest.

Embrace the journey, celebrate the growth, and never lose sight of the profound impact that your commitment to fitness and well-being will have on every aspect of your existence. You are embarking on a sacred odyssey, a journey that will forever shape the person you are destined to become.

The time is now, and the path is yours to claim. Step forward, with confidence and resilience, and let the transformative power of fitness ignite the flame that will illuminate your extraordinary potential, forever.